THE MASTERMINDS OF PLAGUE

A SCIENCE FICTION NOVEL AND A TREATISE ON THE MOST DANGEROUS VIRUSES OF OUR WORLD, INCLUDING THAT OF THE CORONAVIRUS

By Z. Gilead, Ph. D.

Author's Tranquility Press
MARIETTA, GEORGIA

Z. Gilead, Ph. D /Author's Tranquility Press
2706 Station Club Drive SW
Marietta, GA/30060
www.authorstranquilitypress.com

The Masterminds of Plague/ Z. Gilead, Ph. D
Paperback: 978-1-958179-30-7
eBook: 978-1-958179-31-4

About the Author

The author, Dr. Z, Gilead, obtained his M.Sc. degree in Microbiology from the University of Tel Aviv, Israel, and a Ph. D. degree in Virology from the medical school of the University of Pennsylvania in Philadelphia. Later he worked several years as a research scientist in the Institute of Molecular Virology of St. Louis University.

Next, the author returned to his homeland and worked, until his retirement in various start-up companies in the health area.

The author lives in Tel-Aviv, is married and has two sons, two daughters in law and three grandchildren.

Table of Contents

Author's Address

The present novel is a Science Fiction one. But, in addition to its SF genre, it also contains a lot of data on the dangerous viruses of our world, including that of the Coronavirus. It summarizes their histories, life cycles and their clinical impact.

It is also an easy virological guide for lay-people.

I am a retired Virologist and, therefore, I am a little bit out of touch with the current state of virological advances. Therefore, I consulted Wikipedia on some of the scientific data in the book. By assembling the data in one place I am saving my readers a lot of "googling." Besides, even the contributors of the virological data to Wikipedia did not discover the data by their own efforts in the laboratory but gathered it from published papers and scientific summaries.

My novel may seem to be like a virology textbook in some chapters! But it is a "light" textbook that might interest people who do not intend to peruse Virological textbooks in medical school libraries.

And what is the most important, in my novel. I warn scientists not to meddle with viruses by modifying their DNA and RNA!!!

Therefore, pay a few dollars for the book, sit in your favorite armchair, read the Science Fiction story, and concurrently become knowledgeable on the fascinating and the oh so dangerous viruses of our planet.

Introduction

The present novel was written in the time of the Coronavirus pandemic (2020-2022) that swept the entire world, leaving in its wake hundreds of thousands of dead people, invalids, and ruined economies.

In the novel, I want to present myself as a **prophet of doom!**

I need to beg virologists, molecular biologists, and biochemists not to meddle with viruses and not to change the viruses' DNA or RNA!

I am going to offer three Science Fiction novelettes that deal with **fictional** fabricated plagues. I hope that these made-up "prophesies of doom" may serve as warnings for scientists who are currently meddling with the nucleic acid structures of various viruses. These scientists are motivated by scientific curiosity, ambition, and the need to be recognized by peers. But some of them may even want to accommodate the wishes of their warlike masters in totalitarian countries by fashioning biological weapons from viruses. Such scientists may, bring terrible plagues upon their countries' enemies, but also on the entire unsuspecting humanity.

On the Internet, I already see many reports of scientists who "victoriously" describe their virus-modifying successes. When I read these pre-publication entries in Wikipedia, my blood freezes in my veins and I must exclaim: **"Scientists, hands-off! Nature heaps on us, from time to time, enough climate disasters, and plagues. Let us not add to them by creating new ones!"**

I realize that with such public exclamations that are in my novel stand in danger of being labeled as a reactionary and a philistine who does not understand the need for progress in science and the principle of free will, which is one of the most important tenets of a democratic society.

Still, I must act like the elder Cato, a senator in ancient Rome who continuously and strenuously urged his compatriots to promote a third Punic War and to destroy Carthage. In the year 157 BC, he was one of the deputies sent to Carthage to arbitrate between the Carthaginians and Massinissa, king of Numidia. The mission was unsuccessful, and the Roman representatives returned home. However, Cato was so struck by Carthage's growing prosperity that he was convinced that the security of Rome depended on Carthage's complete annihilation.

From that time on, he began concluding his speeches in the Roman Senate, on any topic whatsoever, with the cry, "moreover, I advise to destroy Carthage!" and "Cartago delenda est" (Carthage must be destroyed," in Latin)!

As I indicated in the first lines of the novel, I am a retired virologist. I received an M. Sc. Degree in Microbiology from the University of Tel-Aviv (in 1962) and a pH. D. degree in Virology from the University of Pennsylvania's medical school in Philadelphia (in 1967). After that, I worked as a visiting scientist in the Institute of Molecular Virology of St. Louis University (1967- 1969).

From then on, I joined the Pharmaceutical Industry and worked on subjects that are not related to viruses. Therefore, my virological knowledge is a bit outdated and is partly forgotten... As I already indicated in the introduction, I consulted the Wikipedia on several occasions, and it indeed helped.

As I already indicated, together with the up-to-date virological data, I am also offering three several Science Fiction novelettes on various dangerous viruses that strongly stress the need to refrain from changing the cards that Nature dealt us! I must admit, though, that in some cases, we humans, succeeded in producing good vaccines or therapeutic drugs for various dangerous viruses: Influenza, Coronavirus, HIV, Rabies, Bubonic plague (- "Black death" - caused by the Yersinia pestis bacterium that was spread by the bites of fleas and rats), measles, Rotavirus and Dengue.

Thanks to Dr. Jenner, we abolished the threat of Smallpox virus by vaccination with the related bovine vaccinia virus. However, we are a long way from winning the fight against some existing viruses and those that are currently modified with a complete disregard for Humanity's safety!

Chapter 1

The need to find a true prophet who could warn us of impending plagues

In recent decades, with-and even without-the meddling of scientists, several viruses have jumped from animals to humans and triggered sizable outbreaks that claimed hundreds of thousands of victims. Such a jump of non-infectious animal viruses over species, genera and classes to the human species is called "zoonosis."

The Old Testament describes several fictitious prophets who warned the Jews of impending wars, or famines. In the Middle Ages, Europe had a thousand prophets, but they were false ones, pretenders. In the past, harbingers of new religions: Jesus, Buddha, Muhamad, Baha Ulla, and some others, can be classified as "real" prophets.

For those who believe in prophets with the ability to forecast the future, the most recent popular names are Nostradamus and Baba Vanga.

Michel de Nostredame, usually latinized to Nostradamus, was a French astrologer, physician, and seer, who is best known for his book *"Les Prophéties,"* which was first published in 1555. 'Les Prophéties" ("The prophecies") is a collection of 942 poetic quatrains (four-line verses).

Baba Vanga, also known as" the blind prophet," is one of the more well-known mediums in the world. Even though she died in 1996, some of her predictions are still coming true today.

Her real name was Vangelia Paneva, and she was born in Bulgaria in 1911.

When she was 12 years old, she lost her sight after she was lifted into the air by a tornado and thrown into a nearby field where she was found a few days later with her eyes covered in sand and dust. She made her first predictions a few days after this traumatic event, and legend has it that she developed healing powers and clairvoyance. One of her most significant and noteworthy predictions was the invasion of the Nazis.

A. The prophesies of Nostradamus

The rhymed quatrains of Nostradamus were written in French with a bit of Italian, Greek, Hebrew, and Latin thrown in. He intentionally obscures the quatrains, using symbolism and metaphors, as well as changing last names to proper names, and by swapping, adding, or removing letters. The quatrains were generally ambiguous, but they have been variously interpreted as prophesying important World events.

Many of the prophesies of Nostradamus, when stripped of their obscure "poetic," oracle-like presentations, seem to hit their mark. However, skeptics are quick to point out that Nostradamus' quatrains are so cryptic that they can be interpreted in any number of ways. They suggest that his alleged predictions are nothing more than just misinterpretations or mistranslations. Some of them were even deliberate and may have been fitted and adjusted by their translators to fit major historical events. Other scholars, who have studied his work, believe that Nostradamus had been uncanny in his predictions of some of the most dramatic events of the 20th and previous centuries.

For instance, Nostradamus' believers are claiming that the prophet predicted the appearance of the COVID-19 plague. They point to one of his writings, ("Century 2:53"), which warns: "The great plague of the maritime city will not cease until there be avenged the death of the just' blood, condemned for a price without crime." Although landlocked Wuhan, where the COVID-19 originated, is not a "maritime city," the disease was, possibly traced to seafood markets in a river port near the city of Wuhan. This was enough for the believers to prove a link.

In another quatrain, Nostradamus mentioned a "great plague" in the Italian city of Lucca: "In Lucca it shall come to rain blood and milk, shortly before a change of praetor: Great plague and war, famine and drought shall be made visible." He also warned of a plague striking several cities in Italy: Pau, Verona, Vicenza, Saragossa: "From distant swords lands wet with blood: Very great plague shall come with the great shell."

A plague is also mentioned in relation to France, where many thousands of people have been recently infected and many have died from the COVID-19 plague: "Montauban, Nimes, Avignon and Beziers: Plague, thunder and hail in the wake of Mars: Of Paris bridge, Lyons's wall, Montpellier."

B. The prophesies of Baba Vanga

Lots of the predictions that Baba Vanga made, are expected to be fulfilled in 2020. All of them however are just based on theories from people who believe in clairvoyance and have no scientific foundation.

Drama in Asia

Baba Vanga predicted the famous tsunami of 2004, and if her theories and predictions are to be believed, a much bigger tsunami shall hit parts of Japan, China, Alaska, and Pakistan in 2020. Nearly 400 deaths have already been recorded following an earthquake measuring 7.5 on the Richter scale that hit Indonesia in September.

Putin's life could be in danger

According to Baba Vanga's prophesies, the Russian president Vladimir Putin will be the victim of an assassination attempt and the assassin will be a member of his own security team. Putin admitted that at least four assassination attempts have occurred in the past, but all have failed, and he is currently under the protection of a team of snipers.

Donald Trump will be sick

The president of the United States, Donald Trump, will succumb to an unknown disease. He will suffer from tinnitus, severe nausea, and hearing loss.

President Donald Trump indeed contracted the COVID- 19 plague and recovered after the healing of his physicians.

What will happen after 2020?

By 2023 we would suffer a drastic change on the planet, because the Earth's orbit will change. It will influence the weather, the waters and much of nature, causing great difficulty for humanity to adapt. As a result of this calamity, a change in the ideology of social policy would flourish in the main countries, and by 2076 the entire world would be living under communism.

Nostradamus and Baba Yanga may have been real prophets, or fake ones. However, nowadays, unfortunately, there are no prophets who may warn us of impending dooms.

As for me, I do indeed wish that a real prophet would come that may warn us beforehand of

impending pandemics so that we could work to forestall them!

Chapter 1/1

The Professor meets his team and describes the battle plan for the project

Six young men and women sat in a conference room which was equipped with a slide-projector, projection screen and along with oval conference table with upholstered chairs. The walls of the conference room were lined with rows upon rows of scientific books and journals.

It was obvious that the young men and women did not know each other, as judging by the curious gazes that they directed around. In front of the projection screen, stood a distinguished-looking gentleman of medium weight in his sixties.

He wore a suit and sported a black bow tie and a white shirt. His face reflected kindness and compassion and his blue eyes looked intelligent. He had a beard and was completely bald. When he met new friends and acquaintances, he liked to joke that he woke up one morning and saw that his scalp hair migrated to his chin. This joke always drew hearty guffaws...

The young people had lost their way on coming for the first time to the department, which was the department of Virology and Microbiology in Harvard's Medical School.

They sought their future boss in his office, however, he waited for them in the conference room. On learning of the whereabouts of his team, the professor called his secretary on the phone and asked her to invite the young men and women to the conference /library. When they visited his office on the way to the conference room, the young post-Doctors could see a wall containing several rows of certificates and honorary memberships of scientific societies. The wall also contained several calfskin parchments that cited the prizes that he garnered during his past research. On his desk, they saw a photograph, showing his wife and two sons. A slightly larger silver-framed photograph showed a pretty baby, a granddaughter.

When all the young men and women finally reached the conference room and sat down, their new boss said "Hi there, friends! Welcome to the Department of Virology and Microbiology of Harvard's medical school, in which we shall conduct our research.

As you know from my enrollment advertisements in the "Journal of Virology" and the "Journal of Molecular Biology," my name is Richard Flexner, and I am a full (not fool..., Ha, Ha!) professor in this famous department that you are joining now.

This is the department in whose library we are now convened. I am glad that, obviously, all of you located it. As for me, I was supposed to teach a graduate course of general and medical Virology by Zoom, but since I received a large grant from the CDC (the

Center of Disease Control and Allergy), I requested the chairman of my department to activate a sabbatical year for which I was due next year, and he agreed and found a replacement for me.

Now I want you to get acquainted, but instead of each one you standing-up and declaring his name, I had prepared a slide that will show you who your future colleagues are, and I shall project it in a minute. In my long teaching career, I learned that most people remember material that was presented to them visually. Therefore, watch please a table that presents all of us in our splendor:

Name	Expertise	Previous place of post-doctoring
Jerry Oren	Virology	Department of Virology and Microbiology, Harvard medical school
Josh Kell	Virology	Department of Virology and Microbiology, Harvard medical school
Ayala Gibbons	Virology and Microbiology	Department of Virology and Microbiology, University of California, Los Angeles, Medical school.
Jane Erlanger	Molecular Biology	Department of Molecular Biology, Baylor University School of Medicine
Jim Scuole	Molecular Biology	Department of Molecular Genetics, University of Pennsylvania medical school
Bernardo Bann	Virology and Microbiology	Department of Virology and Microbiology, Johndd Hopkins School Of Medicine

Due to the vagaries of the time in which we find ourselves – the time of the COVID-19 pandemic that left you unemployed I was able to choose a fine collection of brilliant post-doctors – namely you.

I prepared a slide to present the battle plan for our project, which I hope will bring a lot of praise if we succeed.

We are going to work with the recently discovered fearsome variants of the SARS-CoV-2 Coronavirus that are called the British Variant, the "South African variant", and the Indian variant (the Delta). Our purpose is to modify the RNAs of these variants!

As all of you know, the original Coronavirus strain that first infected the entire world, came from the region of Wuhan in China. RNA viruses, also including the Coronaviruses, are more prone to undergo mutations than DNA viruses.

The enhanced infectivity mutations of the recent variants reside in the spike protein of the virus. The spike protein (S) is the target for most of the anti-corona virus vaccines. We shall try to modify the spike protein, so that its attachment to the infected cells will be weak and loose so that it will float in the bloodstream once it disconnects from the cells and will produce antibodies and immune cells against the COVID-19 disease!

You may ask what shall we gain by working hard to modify the Corona variants? Well, – by modifying the variants I hope to make them innocuous – cause them to lose their "pathogenesis" and to be able to induce only a very weakened disease.

This way the host's immune system will be able to produce anti-virus antibodies and immune cells! We shall then disperse the “disarmed,” weakened, innocuous variants in the world and use them as a live vaccine. This may save the World’s populations from the corona scourge.

To produce the weakened, “disarmed” virus in substantial amounts for dispersion around the world we shall also have to find a suitable cell culture that will “agree” to accommodate the weakened virus! This is an overly ambitious program, and, hopefully, the modified variants will become like the well-known case of the Vaccinia virus of cows that immunized very successfully against Smallpox: The bovine Vaccinia Virus is somewhat different from the Smallpox virus but still conferred immunity on those immunized with an ulcer locally on their skin caused by the Vaccinia Virus.

As a result of the many years of vaccination of all human populations with it, Smallpox has disappeared from the surface of the Earth! I am sure that you know that the Vaccinia virus donated its name to a whole newline of Vaccines that confer immunity against Viral, Bacterial and Parasitic diseases.”

Chapter 1/2

Preparations for the Project

Professor Flexner continued:

"For our future work, I have ordered six Class III laminar flow hoods from Labconco Corporation – three hoods for each of our two labs. They should arrive in two weeks' time.

These class III laminar flow hoods have the highest level of safety and create an air-tight environment for work with dangerous materials and infectious human pathogens. In the meantime, you and I shall have to be immunized with the FDA-approved Pfizer's or Moderna's vaccines. They induce immunity even against the fearsome American, South African, British, and Indian variants. We shall be able to start the actual lab work a week after the second injection of the vaccine. In addition, we shall also wear the best protective uniforms and equipment that money can buy.

Until that time, you will have to do a lot of scientific reading...I expect all of you to come to the start of our lab work brimming with ideas and knowledge of all the recent scientific technics.

In the new Minus 70 degrees Revco freezers that I had purchased for our project, there are already stored ampules of all the very infective Variants of the coronavirus that our sponsor – the WHO sent me.

I also have mice, hamsters, minks, and monkeys in a sterile protected animal house. This will allow us to infect the animals with the zoonotic[1]) strains and cultivate the viruses for our mRNA modification attempts.

Our instrumentation department contains the most modern DNA-, RNA and Protein synthesizers and analyzers, and you can use them freely under the supervision of their technicians.

Recently we have introduced to our Instrumentation department the excellent and amazingly fast Next-generation sequencing (NGS) of RNA. This method provides an effective, unbiased way to identify new coronavirus strains and other pathogens without prior knowledge of organisms. Growing concern over fast-spreading, novel variants of the SARS-CoV-2 coronavirus, such as the B.1.1.7 strain [UK] and B1.351 strain (S. Africa), and the Delta strain highlights the need for more sequencing to detect mutations quickly and prevent the spread of new strains. Sequencing was used to identify the novel coronavirus causing COVID-19 (SARS-CoV-2) early in the outbreak. NGS continues to provide public health officials, vaccine and drug developers, and researchers with critical evidence, allowing labs to:

- To quickly track the transmission routes of the virus globally.

---

[1] *Zoonotic - a disease that can be transmitted to humans from animals.*

- Detect mutations quickly to prevent the spread of new variants.
- Identify viral mutations that can avoid detection by established molecular diagnostic assays.
- Identify viral mutations that can affect vaccine potency.
- Screen drugs for possible COVID-19 therapeutics
- Identify and characterize respiratory co-infections and antimicrobial resistance alleles)[2].

Our Microbiological plus Molecular Genetics and Virology department are quite famous for their many scientific advances, and we have several Nobel laureate prize winners among our academic ranks. A post-doctoral work in our department can gain you several plus points in the future job market after Corona.

Professor Flexner continued: "Please be advised that there are several scientific groups that are working on the same project that we intend to study. I hope, for the sake of Humanity, that they will succeed. But even more so I hope that we shall be the ones to succeed before everybody else...Therefore, let us "gird up our loins" and go on to solve the COVID-19 problem!"

---

[2] *Alleles- An allele is an alternative form of a gene (one member of a pair) that is located at a specific position on a specific chromosome. These DNA codings determine distinct traits that can be passed on from parents to offspring through sexual reproduction.*

Then Professor Flexner added: "Dear colleagues, each one of you will get a room in the students' dormitory which is mostly unoccupied now because of the Corona. It is still cleaned, and it will also be supplied weekly with clean linen and towels. Jerry Oren and Josh Kell, my Post-Docs whom I tutor, already live there with their girlfriends. You can ask them for details about their experiences.

In addition, you can dine in the University's dining hall which is still open. This way you will be able to work without daily hassles and will also be able to save your salaries which will be 84,000 Dollars for the first year, and slightly higher for the second year, should there be one."

Here Bernardo raised his hand, interrupting the flow of Professor Flexner's talk. The professor stopped and allowed Bernardo to pose his urgent question. Bernardo said: "Sir, thank you for all the goodies that you arranged for us, including the generous salary! However, I still have a favor to ask from you: May I bring my girlfriend to the dormitory with me? We have been together for 3 years. It will be difficult for me to stay here apart

From her! We intended to rent an apartment in the city, but perhaps you could allow her to live with me in the dormitory?"

Professor Flexner answered: "Bernardo, by all means! I want to keep you happy and efficient! In addition, please do not 'sir" me! We shall use only forenames among us since all of us are colleagues now!" Here Jim popped up and said: "Richard, I, too would like to bring my fiancé with me to the dormitory. Is that also Okay with you?"

The professor answered: "Why Jim, most certainly! I shall tell my secretary Agnes to pick family apartments with larger bathrooms for you and for Bernardo and your girlfriends!"

Then Jane also joined her friends with a "me too," Richard pretended to be amazed and said: "Hey Jane, nobody is trying to molest you sexually! Why do you bring this feminine fighting slogan into our midst" Jane smiled and said that she has a fiancé who is a Ph. D., and he is currently unemployed, He remained at Baylor University where both had worked before she applied to work for with Flexner. Jane continued: "Richard, since you are so generous, can I bring also my fiancé?" Richard immediately acceded also to her request. Then Richard said: "One of the first things that I did when I obtained the grant, was to hire a secretary who will help you with your lodging in the students' dormitory, dining in the dining hall, and will arrange for you employee identity cards and all other official and unofficial needs.

To hire her, I applied to the almost defunct employment office of the University, and they sent me several available secretaries for interviews. These had lost their jobs in various departments because of the Corona.

I chose an elderly lady by the name of Agnes Merriweather who impressed me with her references. I hired her also because I wanted to save her from unemployment...

Agnes quickly prepared for all of us a fully equipped office with all sorts of communication devices. You will be able to communicate on both personal and on scientific matters with the entire world. I consider her a vital part of our small organization.

We also have in the department a large kitchen that is not used. My scientific colleagues in the department who still teach or do research, go to the dining hall, or to a cafeteria that is still open. With the Dean's permission and, because of a handsome donation from my grant to the department, I obtained the kitchen for our sole use, and I also hired a cook. She will fulfill your requests for nourishment, in addition to the dining hall, from 11:00 to 20:00 at night." Then, Richard added: "Remember that you have at present four weeks free time. Use it to settle various personal matters and do not forget to use the libraries in your previous institutions!

You are invited now to examine both of our labs and the Department's equipment Annex. It is full to the brim with the most modern scientific equipment and has two experienced technicians to help you. I shall see you again in four weeks' time. If you stay today a few more hours at the end of our meeting, Agnes will supply you then, or when you come back in four weeks' time, with personnel identity cards. These will serve you for entrance and all your needs in the department, including the entrance to the dining hall. She also has permission from the Dean to show you rooms in the students' dormitory to choose from. Please tell her also your girlfriends,' and boyfriend' names for their identity cards."

Finally, the young men and women bid farewell to their older colleague-boss Professor Flexner and went to the cafeteria to chat and to wait for Agnes. Four weeks after the team's first meeting with Professor Flexner, the men and women came back eagerly to start their research.

Richard welcomed them warmly, asked them to choose a lab from the two Project's labs and immediately came to business. He said: "As you saw in my famous personnel chart, two of our group, Jerry Oren and Josh Kell were fortunate enough to work as post-Docs in my lab...! Ha, Ha!

Jerry worked under my tutelage on the genetic aspects of the coronavirus and his knowledge had expanded, and by now well exceeds mine! Josh became an expert on the life cycle of the COVID-19 virus, its nucleic acid and its proteins and he will enlighten us after Jerry's talk. Right now, we are strangers to each other. However, I know that once we shall start our work and dine together, we shall get more familiar with each other.

You will work either alone, or in collaboration with one, two or more of us, but remember that we shall not compete, but must co-operate! Please choose the lab that catches your fancy and a workbench in that lab. You can also choose your companion(s) to cooperate with. Note that no choice is iron-clad. You will be able to change places when you may want to change partners. Every Tuesday- and Friday morning we shall meet at 8:00 for one hour of brainstorming. That is all. If you do not have any pressing questions, go to your labs and God bless!"

THEN THE PROFESSOR SAID TO OUR READERS:

Dear readers!

The following chapters contain difficult scientific data. I have inserted many footnotes that explain difficult terms that need to be clarified. Sometimes even these footnotes may not be sufficient. In this case, try at least to absorb the essence and aroma of the science without any additional digging....

Chapter 1/3

Jerry describes the Wuhan Strain and its variants

At the end of four weeks, the post-docs came back to the department, eager to start working. Professor Flexner assembled them in the conference room/library, welcomed them, and started immediately to indoctrinate them.

He addressed Jery and said: "Jerry, my wise epidemiologist, would you please enlighten the team from your vast store of Corona lore? the chair is yours, or perhaps you would rather stand up?"

Jerry, stood up, went to the front of the conference room, near the projection screen, and said:

"Hi fellas! Here comes my excellent exposition...If you have any questions, I shall answer them at the end of my narration.

I realize that the virologists among us know all, or most of what I am going to describe, so that my "wise" words will be mostly directed at the Molecular geneticists among us!

As all of you know, Coronaviruses are a group of related RNA viruses that cause disease in mammals and birds. They cause in them respiratory tract infections that can range from mild to lethal. In rare cases, the Coronaviruses become what scientists call "zoonotic," meaning they can be transmitted from animals to humans and cause profoundly serious respiratory and other terrible body symptoms.

All the coronaviruses denoted as "CoV" are a type of retrovirus pseudo-type (they imitate retroviruses like HIV in their mode of their nucleic acid replication).

RNA viruses mutate very often, and SARS-Cov-2 is no exception. I want to describe to you the mutants of the SARS-Cov-2, otherwise also known as COVID-19 virus. It is true that all knowledgeable people in the world are already acquainted with the frightful progression of the mutants (almost each one of the newer variants is more dangerous than the previous ones). Still, I think that we ought to know as much as possible on our enemies. The very first mutant, the Wuhan variant, originated, apparently, from bats that are bountiful in several regions of the Republic of China. It may have passed from bats through an intermediate animal (possibly a Pangolin[3]) with a non-zoonotic corona of its own, and because of a chance event of genetic recombination – the hybrid virus become zoonotic and infected humans.

However, there are scientists that support another opinion than that of the Pangolin recombination theory and propose that the mutant was engineered in a virological lab in Wuhan, China. The purpose of the putative Wuhan genetic engineering presumably

---

[3] *Pangolin - an African and Asian mammal that has a body covered with horny overlapping scales, a small head with an elongated snout, a long sticky tongue for catching ants and termites, and a tapering tail. Also called scaly anteater.*

intended to modify bat viruses with the wish to study how to prevent them from infecting humans during mutations, or to determine what pharmaceutical drugs will kill them, in case it should happen. Unfortunately, the mutant became zoonotic and perhaps infected a lab person by accident, so he became "infected person No. 1" and spread the virus further. I must say, though, that this idea had been discredited by many scientists, and the pangolin idea remained, although with a question mark still attached to it....

The SARS Cov-2 causes the COVID-19 disease whose symptoms are profoundly serious: respiratory, cardiac, and liver damage symptoms, extreme weakness, elevated temperature and finally death in a certain percent of young grown-up and old people. Persons who suffer from background ailments are more vulnerable. Because it affects the lungs, many patients need to be sedated and ventilated. COVID-19 may also cause serious sequelae in some "cured" people that take months to recover, and not even then. Many infected patients, and more so children, are asymptomatic – that is, they may not display any symptoms, but they can infect other people.

Since RNA viruses mutate often, this has cast a shadow of doubt on the current vaccines. The vaccines may fail to protect against the more advanced mutations. Note that mutants should be more correctly named variants, as I shall soon describe. Luckily, the scientists of Pfizer declared that their vaccine is effective against all the variants known today. In addition, the said that the vaccine confers immunity for the duration of one year. They modified this duration later to 4-6 months.

Let me list now the current known variants. Please God that no more variants will be added to the list. Unfortunately, when COVID-19 faces an existence pressure, it mutates even more.

Also, when the virus infects a person with a weakened immune system, such as a cancer patient, it lingers for many weeks in the patient without killing him. During the stay, it has enough time to mutate...

The terms **"strain,"** **"variant"** and **"mutant"** are often, mistakenly, used interchangeably. So, what exactly is the difference between a variant, strain, and mutation?

The term **"strain"** is only appropriate when referring to SARS-Cov-2. It is since it is the only one strain of the wider Beta Coronavirideae family. This family includes in addition to the SARS Cov-2, the zoonotic and dangerous severe acute respiratory syndrome virus (SARS), and the Middle East Respiratory Syndrome virus (MERS) strains and some non-zoonotic strains that I will not list. I will soon describe these zoonotic strains. The Viruses of the Linnean [4]) family that I will describe here, are strains. The strains easily mutate, and the resulting progeny are called **variants.**

What is a **mutation**? Mutation is the process by which a strain can make new variants. In the virus, and all organisms, in one or more places, one nucleotide or more in the DNA or RNA are deleted and/or replaced by one or more additional nucleotides. This may sound frightening to many millions of already infected and uninfected persons – but we, the scientists, know that it is a "normal" event in the life of all organisms in Nature."

The three pandemic-causing zoonotic strains

Jerry continued:" I already mentioned the three dangerous Coronavirideae strains that I want you to meet.

1) **Severe Acute Respiratory Syndrome (SARS).** The SARS virus is a coronavirus that can cause severe symptoms. To show that the SARS virus belongs to the same family as the SARS-Cov-2 and the MERS VIRUS that I shall soon describe, it is called SARS-Cov without the number "2" of the COVID-19 strain. It came in 2002-2004 from the Guangdong province in southern China where it was identified in 2003. It causes respiratory problems but also diarrhea, fatigue,

---

[4] *Linnean–Linnaeus-A Swedish botanist, zoologist, taxonomist, and physician who formalized binomial nomenclature, the modern system of naming organisms.)*

shortness of breath, respiratory distress, and kidney failure. Depending on the patient's age, the death rate with SARS ranged from 0-50% of the cases, with older people being the most vulnerable. Scientists suspect that a passage of a bat virus in civet cats[5]) caused zoonosis.

2) **The Middle East Respiratory Syndrome (MERS)**. It was first reported in the Arabian desert in 2012and caused serious respiratory problems. Three to four out of every 10 patients who were unlucky enough to be infected with the MERS virus died. Scientists think that the MERS virus originated in camels.

3) **The third zoonotic strain is SARS-Cov-2**. As everybody in our poor globe heard by now, that strain causes the current COVID-19 Pandemic. It is thought to be milder than MERS and SARS, but it takes longer to develop symptoms. This late development of symptoms is very disadvantageous since humans become carriers of infection when they are still without any symptoms. So far, around 15% to 20% of cases become severe, requiring artificial respiration in the hospital or even connection to an ECMO[6]) instrument. Luckily, the highly infectious Delta

---

[5] *Civet cats-A civet is a small, lean, mostly nocturnal mammal native to tropical Asia and Africa, especially the tropical forests. The term civet applies to over a dozen different mammal species.)*

[6] *ECMO instrument - Extracorporeal membrane oxygenation (ECMO), is an extracorporeal (outside the body) technique of providing prolonged cardiac and respiratory support to persons whose heart and lungs are unable to provide an adequate amount of gas exchange or perfusion to sustain life. The technology for ECMO is derived from cardiopulmonary bypass*

variant causes only a small number of severe cases, although it also infects persons who were immunized with 2 injections of an RNA vaccine. As I already told you, its symptoms are remarkably like those of MERS and SARS-Coc-2."

"Now I want to list the variants of the SARS-Cov-2",

Jerry said. He wrote the names of the variants of the COVID-19 on the screen of the conference/library and proceeded to describe them: "With the appearance of the new highly infective variants of SARS-Cov-2, physicians are faced with terrible symptoms that leave them perplexed and stymied. They strive to treat these symptoms but are only partly successful. In this respect, the corona pandemic is different from other plagues!

The Chinese, in whose Wuhan region this variant appeared, are blamed for not informing the world early enough on its existence. They quickly built many field hospitals for their own citizens at the very start of the pandemic and failed to nip the pandemic in the bud, or to notify the world early enough of its existence!

Let me now list the variants of the Wuhan strain that started the Pandemic:

1. The Wuhan strain of the COVID-19: A scientist named Shi Zhengli from the Wuhan Institute of Virology, published a paper saying that the novel worldwide spreading coronavirus (COVID-19) was 96 percent identical to a bat virus, named by her as

RATG13. She implied that the COVID-19 was derived naturally from a bat virus, perhaps through recombination in a second animal that harbored another strain of coronavirus as I already mentioned.

2. "Variant 5": This is a variant which arose in minks that were infected by their human tenders. The "Variant 5" of the OVID-19 is more infective than the Wuhan variant but is not more lethal. It can be neutralized by the antibodies elicited by the current mRNA vaccines.

Denmark had taken a drastic step of culling millions of minks, following the emergence of the variant 5. European citizens were not allowed by their governments to enter Denmark. Luckily, this variant did not spread much and has been supplanted by more infectious ones.

3. The British Variant: This mutant possesses the designation D614G. This designation indicates that the letter code D (Aspartic acid) in the Wuhan variant mutated into G (Glycine). It possesses also other 23 non-dangerous mutations that were not present in the original Wuhan strain. Scientists hypothesized that it survived several months in a person with an impaired immune system and during that time the mass of virions in that person developed the mutations. Anyway, as I already told you, RNA viruses mutate quickly and faster than DNA viruses. It is quite possible that the Brazilian and South African variants, which I shall soon describe, also passed through a person with a weak immune system.

The British (ALPHA) variants with its D614G mutation spread more quickly than the original Wuhan strain and in addition, are more lethal. It was first detected in farmworkers in Catalonia and Aragon. It is responsible for 90 percent of new infections in Spain in June and has spread across Europe because of tourists visiting the country. When the British variant had come from Spain, it was called "VOC 202012/01". Now it has a new designation of B.1.1.7. This variant has triggered a second, widespread wave of infection in the UK and from there it became the most prevalent mutant in quite a few countries. Luckily, Pfizer's scientists found out recently that their vaccine also works against the British variant.

The British variant made its first highly infectious "debut" in London and in many other areas in Kent – before it migrated to many other countries in Europe, as well as to other continents. In June-July of 2021 it was supplanted by the highly infectious Indian (DELTA) variant.

4. Very recently, a new variant appeared in South Africa. It has been originally designated as 501.V2 (OMICRON) and now it has the designation of B.1. 351. It is very infectious and spreads fast in the population. Its RNA sequence is different from that of the earlier variants, and it caused a great concern that the current RNA vaccines may not be able to neutralize it. However, a scientist who helped in the development of the AstraZeneca/Oxford vaccine, has

said that the current vaccines could be effective even against this highly infectious variant.

5. A new variant has been added to the "treasury of plagues." It started in Brazil and is designated P.1. (ZETA, GAMMA) Apparently, the use of successful vaccines caused the COVID-19 to mutate at an even faster rate.

Each of these last 3 variants, The British, the South African and the Brazilian variants contain in their viral RNA unique mutation(s) that differed from the other two. However, all 3 variants have one thing in common – they are 6-8- times more infectious than the Wuhan strain. This enhanced infectivity is caused in all 3 variants by the D614Gmutation that I mentioned previously.

6. A worrying new variant appeared in New York City, in California and elsewhere in the Northeast of the USA. Cases of this variant, named B.1.526, (EPSILON, IOTA) have now spread across all states in the US. It bears a unique set of spike mutations. I forgot to mention that all the dangerous mutations that I mentioned till now, occur in the RNA region of the spikes that I will soon describe).

There are two versions of the New York variant. Both are called B.1.526 variants for now. One version carries the E484K mutation, which was independently found also in the Brazilian and the South African variants. Scientists are afraid that this mutation may reduce the effectiveness of current vaccines. The other version has a S477N mutation which may act like a "tour-guide" for COVID-19 to infect human cells, optimizing the binding process and increasing infection rates.

7. It appears that our troubles are not yet over! An additional variant appeared in India. It is officially called B.1.617 and "DELTA." It was first identified in March and has spread to many countries all over the world. It is the first variant that carries mutations in 2 separate places of the spike. I have already indicated that it is extremely infectious, it appears also in previously immunized people but luckily, it is less virulent than many other variants. After two years, COVID-19 remains mysterious. This is mainly because of the case rate of infection with the Delta variant. Currently, Austria, Germany, France, Italy, the UK, Slovakia Hungary, Poland, and the Netherlands carry a high caseload of infected persons. Japan, on the other hand, has seen a case rate which is falling to historical low – currently the case rate is 50 daily cases. At this same time, the US reports a daily average of more than a thousand cases daily.

What can be the reason for this phenomenon? Geneticists propose that the Japanese Delta variant first outcompeted all earlier variants and then it mutated to a faulty virus unable to copy itself efficiently. As a result, it is headed towards extinction, just like the SARS outbreak in 2004. Other scientists attribute the decrease in case of rate to the high immunity percent in Japan – 76%. Moreover, the

Japanese are used to wearing face masks as they did even before the corona.

8. A reigning new mutant appeared in South Africa and spread to the entire world which WHO scientists have named as OMICRON. It carries over 50 mutations and it is extremely infectious. Luckily, its disease proved to be mild and can be even treated at home if it is in immunized people. It has a high infectivity index that is greater than1 (several persons who are in proximity to a diagnosed person get infected, and not just one of the persons as in a virus with an **infectivity coefficient** of 1.0). The Omicron variant is immune to the RNA vaccines and infects also immunized people but the disease that appears is mild and the infected patients can be treated at home. However, nonimmunized persons contract a severe disease, need to be hospitalized and a certain percent of them dies! The symptoms of an infected person disappear after a short while in immunized persons and take much longer to disappear in nonimmunized persons. However, the virus may cause the appearance of the so-called LONG COVID). This condition is not unique just to Omicron and happens also in the earlier variants such as Alpha to Delta (I must admit that I failed to discuss the LONG COVID condition when I described the earlier mutants...) Long Covid, (it is not clear how long it takes) is a completely different entity than a "regular infection." It is a chronic disease with grave symptoms that differ from person to person, but include the condition of

the production of self-antibodies against the tissues of the patient which cause the awakening of several long-gone viruses and damage to the brain, alimentary tract, lymph nodes, etc. The Long Covid has an incidence of 10-30 % with varying degree of severity.

9. And if the damage caused by OMICRON is not enough, there exists now a new variant called BA2, which appears to possess an even greater infectivity, but not greater morbidity than that of Omicron. In vaccinated people it gives rise to a mild disease like Omicron.

Chapter 1/4

Tests for an infection with COVID-19

Here Jerry stopped his talk for a few seconds, drank some water and then continued; "Now I want to describe to you an especially important subject: the tests for virus infectivity.

Tests for infection with COVID-19

It is common knowledge in the whole suffering world that there are quite a few tests to determine infection I shall list the types of tests used. The tests belong to 2 main groups:

1. Molecular tests (measuring the presence of viral RNA), and
2. Serological tests for the presence of the COVID-19's antibodies and COVID-19's antigen.

When, and if, we develop our "disarmed mutant," following a world-wide dispersion of our presumably successful disarmed mutant, we shall have to recommend what test will best detect the infection.

1. Molecular tests

A Molecular test for the presence of viral RNA is used to accurately diagnose a current infection with the virus. These molecular tests are the gold standard of all types of tests. They are the most accurate, but time-consuming tests. They are represented by the Nucleic Acid Amplification Tests (NAATs) that I will describe now and center on the viral RNA. NAAT tests are dependent upon a method that multiplies the few copies of viral RNA present in a patients' test specimen into many copies. At present, most NAAT tests use an amplification method called Reverse Transcriptase[7]) polymerase chain reaction (RT PCR).

This test uses small segments of DNA, called "primers," which pick out the DNA that was originally synthesized on the template of the viral RNA in the test samples with the reverse transcriptase. PCR instruments then automatically replicate this DNA by in repeated cycles of heating and cooling. During each cycle, the number of copies of the targeted nucleic acid, doubles by the action of the heat-stable DNA polymerase. From a few original copies, it can generate up to a billion new copies to make the virus easier to see in the final detection step which is electrophoresis in agar.

NAAT tests are molecular diagnostics tests against many RNA gene targets. The patients' samples for the NAAT test are respiratory specimens collected from individuals after a "window period" of up to 5 days after exposure during which corona cannot be detected. However, false negative NAAT results can

---

[7] *Reverse transcriptase - A reverse transcriptase (RT) is an enzyme used to generate complementary DNA (DNA) from an RNA template, a process termed reverse transcription. It is used in the PCR with which it is possible to generate thousands to millions of copies of a particular section of DNA from an exceedingly small amount of DNA.*

also occur even after this 5-day window. Therefore, to exclude SARS-CoV-2 infection - a repeat testing several days later must be used to confirm or rule out infection.

COVID-19 poses several diagnostic challenges, including potentially different shedding of virus along the breathing ways. However, due to the high specificity of NAAT, a positive result in a NAAT of an upper respiratory tract sample is enough to diagnose corona.

The respiratory test samples are nasopharyngeal swab, sputum (coughed up material), throat swabs, and deep airway material collected via a suction catheter or saliva. The test samples are treated with certain chemicals that allow nucleic acids (RNA) to be extracted.

2. Serological tests

I. Antigen tests. An Antigen test measures whether there is a current infection in the tested patient by detecting the presence of the viral proteins (= antigen, generally spike protein). The tests are rapid (take up to 20-30 minutes to supply a result) but they are not as sensitive as the molecular PCR-based tests. These "While-you-wait" tests that detect the spike proteins in sputum are better at diagnosing the disease in patients with symptoms than in those without symptoms.

A recent analysis found that on average, "antigen tests" correctly identified 72 percent of symptomatic COVID-19 cases but only 58 per cent of cases in people devoid of symptoms.

Antigen tests are Lateral flow tests, also known as lateral flow immune chromatographic assays or rapid tests. They use simple devices intended to detect the presence of a target substance (in this case-coronavirus spike proteins).

In these tests, corona virus **antibodies** (native or synthetically produces) are absorbed to a Nitro-Cellulose paper or other absorbents) on one hand, and chemically treated sputum samples (to liberate the spike proteins of the virions in them) are flowed laterally along an absorbent. These tests are widely used in medical diagnostics for home testing, or laboratory use. An example of such tests is the home pregnancy test that detects a certain fertility hormone in laterally flowed urine. These tests are simple, economic, and show results in around 10 to 30 minutes.

Many lab-based applications increase the sensitivity of simple lateral flow tests by employing additional dedicated equipment. In all these tests the detection is with horse radish peroxidase that is linked to the reactants.

II. <u>Antibody tests</u> - In essence, these tests run the

liquid sample of blood or plasma or serum) along the **surface of a pad containing absorbed spike proteins** that show a visual positive stain signal. The pads are based on a series of capillary beds, such as pieces of porous paper, micro-structured polymer, or sintered polymer. Each of these pads has the capacity to transport fluids (e.g., serum, blood, plasma), The sample pad acts as a sponge and holds an excess of laterally flowing patient fluid (blood, serum, plasma). Once soaked, the patient fluids flow to the second conjugate pad in which the manufacturer has stored freeze-dried bio-active particles called conjugates in a salt-sugar matrix. The conjugate pad contains all the reagents required for an optimized chemical reaction between the target molecule (e.g., an antigen in the blood, serum, plasma) and its chemical partner (e.g., antibody), that had been immobilized on the pad's surface. A positive test line shows color ed line as in pregnancy tests. After passing these reaction zone, the fluid enters the final porous material, the wick, which simply acts as a waste container.

III. Antibody Tests by ELISA - This second type of antibody tests show whether someone at present, or at some time in the past, had the disease. They are less useful for diagnosing current infections because antibodies may not develop for weeks after infection. Because SARS- CoV-2 transmission occurs days after exposure (and before the onset of symptoms) there is an urgent need for frequent surveillance and rapid availability of results. As an example, out of several such tests, I want to describe to you The Rapid Antibody test which is the Rapid ELISA test (Enzyme-Linked Immunosorbent Assay) called VITROS which is a product of Orto Clinics. In this test, ELISA plates, which are plastic blocks containing 8×12 wells (holes) are coated with a viral protein (either the spike protein or the envelope [E] proteins). I am sure that Josh will describe these viral proteins later.

Then plasma samples from infected patients that may contain COVID-19 antibodies (mostly IgM or IgG), and uninfected persons are incubated with the **viral protein "coat"** in the plates, allowing any NON-immune globulins to be removed by washing, whereas anti-COVID-19 antibody, (IgG or IgM) are bound to the plates (through the coated virus proteins) and are detected by the addition of HRP[8])-conjugated anti

---

[8] *HRP - The enzyme horseradish peroxidase (HRP), found in the roots of horseradish, is used extensively in biochemistry applications. It is a metalloenzyme with many isoforms, of which the most studied type is C. It catalyzes the oxidation of various organic substrates by hydrogen peroxide. The substrate of the enzyme that is most used is DAB. Dab is DAB (3,3'-Diaminobenzidine)is a water-soluble, chromogenic substrate of horseradish peroxidase (HRP), a common label conjugated to antibodies. HRP catalyzes the oxidation of DAB by hydrogen peroxide. The result is a brown precipitate that localizes to the sites of HRP-bound antibodies.*

total or IgG antibodies. Detection is by the addition of HRP substrate DAB which stains the positive anti COVID-19 (total or IgG antibodies in the positive wells).

The test has a high throughput which allows the testing of 130 samples per hour and yields the results of total and IgG antibodies. At the end of the test, the results of the plates are read with a specially designed computing ELISA reading instrument.

IgM and IgG antibodies are found even as early as the fourth day after symptom onset, but higher levels occur only in the second and third week of illness.

Typically, most antibodies are produced against the most abundant protein of the virus - the Nucleocapsid (NC). Therefore, tests that detect antibodies to NC would be the most sensitive. However, the receptor-binding domain of the Spike protein (RBD-S) is the one that attaches to the host cell, and, therefore, antibodies to RBD-S would be more specific and are expected to be neutralizing.

Rapid tests for the detection of antibodies have been widely developed and marketed and are of variable quality. Many manufacturers do not reveal the nature of antigens used to coat plates. These tests are purely qualitative in nature and can only indicate the presence or absence of SARS-CoV-2 antibodies and not their concentration.

The long-term persistence and duration of protection conferred by neutralizing antibodies remain unknown. Pfizer says that the first and second immunization injections confer 4-6 months' immunity while booster third and fourth injection confer longer immunity.

How does COVID-19 exert its damage?

Jerry continued: "The mechanism that COVID-19 causes damage to the human body is the following:

COVID-19 antigens are presented to tissue residing antigen-presenting cells (APCs) such as macrophages, which in turn produce a range of inflammatory cytokines[9]). Ultimately, these cytokines cause the proliferation of an enhanced, unbalanced, and devastating inflammatory response in the host ("cytokine storm") which causes heavy damage to most critical organs!

The factors that affect the virus pathogenesis in patients with COVID-19, are background cardiovascular, cerebrovascular diseases, as well as diabetes. There are several additional abnormalities that exacerbate the disease, and these are cellular immune deficiency, coagulation activation, myocardial injury, hepatic and kidney injury, and secondary bacterial infection. In most cases of severe disease and death, lymphopenia (decreased lymphocyte concentration) and sustained inflammation have been recorded. Notably, these

---

[9] *Cytokines- "cytokines" is an umbrella term that includes all kinds of substances. There are specific names given to cytokines based on either the type of cell that makes them or the action they have in the body: The immune system is complex—several types of immune cells and proteins do different jobs. Cytokines are among those proteins.*

observations in COVID-19 patients are like those patients who suffered from severe acute respiratory syndrome (SARS) during the 2003 epidemic. There may be an identical biological mechanism behind these anomalies."

Chapter 1/5

Anti-COVID-19 vaccines

Then Jerry added: "Finally, I want to add some words on the Anti- COVID 19's vaccines: Many companies worked feverishly to develop a vaccine which will neutralize the COVID-19's attachment protein (Spike Proteins). Currently, four companies had advanced enough in their clinical trials, and received FDA'S approval. These are Pfizer with its German collaborator BioNTech, Moderna, (both are RNA vaccines). The British AstraZeneca Oxford and the American Johnson and Johnson offered a Chimpanzee Flu or Chimpanzee Cold viruses that contains the COVID-19's replicated double stranded DNA integrated into the DNA of the carrier virus. On entering a cell, this double stranded DNA is transcribed into the mRNA of the COVID-19 and translates the viral structural proteins (S, M, N, and E) which either I or Josh will soon describe.

Unfortunately, Both AstraZeneca's and Johnson and Johnson's vaccines were found to possess a side-effect, although in an exceptionally low frequency. This side-effect is the appearance of blood clots in the circulation. Several countries decided to limit the use of these two vaccines to certain age groups only.

The four vaccines that I described above are expensive and, in fact, intended for rich countries.

The Chinese are offering poor or less rich countries their own vaccines that is produced mainly by Sinovac and Sinopharm companies. These two Chinese companies offer their vaccines either cheaply or gratis.

This act helps them to penetrate new markets. Sinovac Biotech grows the virus in cell cultures and then kills the virions with a chemical called Beta Propiolactone- that binds to the viral mRNA. The vaccine is called CoronaVac. Sinopharm uses live attenuated virions that underwent genetic engineering and is like the vaccines of oral polio, measles, rotavirus, and yellow fever.

The mRNA vaccines of Pfizer and Moderna are a novel technology, where the viral mRNA - once it gets into the cell-instructs the body's cells to make copies of the Spike and other proteins of the virus and produce antibodies and immune cells against them.

The positive sense mRNA of the Pfizer's and Moderna's vaccines is an isolated mRNA or apart thereof. When it gets into an infected cell, it is translated. Their technic of the production of the viral mRNA was not described. Possibly it used automatic RNA synthesizers. At any rate, as I already described, the vaccine contains a large part or whole single-stranded positive sense mRNA (like the RNA of a normal infecting virus).

Using the cell's tRNA and ribosomes, the mRNA, including the spike proteins, is translated. The translated viral proteins migrate to the cell's surface and are presented to the body's immune mechanisms and induce the synthesis of antibodies and immune white cells which confer immunity to the vaccinated persons.

The Pfizer BioNTech COVID-19 vaccine and Moderna's vaccines do not contain any live virus but mRNA and excipients[10]) and an artificially made lipid nanoparticle envelope. A word on the safety of the novel RNA vaccines that worried some people: Once translated, the mRNA of the vaccines is digested by the host's enzymes. It is never processed into DNA – a situation that could affect the DNA genome and cause serious side effects and genetic problems. This is because the infected cell does not possess an RNA-dependent DNA polymerase.

Therefore, the mRNA vaccine cannot produce any viral DNA which could affect the cell DNA genetically. Therefore, RNA vaccines are completely safe! The mRNA vaccines (of both Pfizer and Moderna) are injected in two doses, 3weeks apart.

The second injection re-enforces the first injection because of immune memory B cells that were induced by the first injection. Pfizer says it uses four different lipids to produce the nanoparticles for the envelope in a "defined ratio."

---

[10] *Excipient - an inactive substance that serves as the vehicle or medium for a drug or other active substance.*

One ingredient in the formulation of Pfizer's vaccine is known. That is ALC-0315 which is the primary ingredient. That is because it is ionizable— it can be given a positive charge, and since the RNA has a negative one, they stick together.

The other lipids, one of which is the molecule of cholesterol, are liposomes. They are "helpers" that give structural integrity to the nanoparticles or stop them from clumping. During manufacturing, the RNA and the lipids are stirred into a bubbly mix. To enter the cell to begin the process, the liposomes utilize HLA[11]) proteins on the infected cell membrane.

The spike mRNA gene sequence can be changed in small ways for better performance by swapping nucleotide letters in the mRNA. Pfizer has not said exactly what sequence it is using, or what modified nucleosides. That, of course, is Pfizer's prerogative as a commercial company.

The Pfizer vaccine contains four salts, one of which is ordinary chart salt. Together, these salts are better known as phosphate-buffered saline, or PBS, a quite common ingredient that keeps the pH, or acidity, of the vaccine close to that of a person's body.

---

[11] *HLA - The human leukocyte antigen (HLA) system or complex is a group of related proteins that are encoded by the major histocompatibility complex (MHC) gene complex in humans. These cell-surface proteins are responsible for the regulation of the immune cells system in humans.*

The vaccine also contains plain sugar (sucrose). It is acting here as a cryoprotectant to safeguard the nanoparticles when they are frozen and stop them from sticking together.

Pfizer's company and researchers from the University of Texas Medical Branch, carried out laboratory tests on different COVID-19 variants, including the British, the Brazilian and the South African ones and they have found that their vaccine confers immunity also against these dangerous variants.

As I already told you, Pfizer BioNTech announced that their vaccine is good for 5-6 months in the term of the presence of antibodies and their activity. After this period, a second injection must be given that is also good for 5-6 months and after that a third and even a fourth injections which are called "Boosters," must be given to immune-challenged and old people and those with health risks.

This may mean that a third and a fourth injection of the current vaccine, or one or two of a new vaccine, will be needed.

Then Jerry added: "Just recently, an article appeared in the New-York Times that wrote the following: 'In the initial stages of the COVID-19's outbreaks there existed the hope that the world will reach one day a state of 'Herd Immunity"– the point where there will not be enough people that can be infected easily.

Despite these hopes, more than two years passed since the start of the Pandemic and third, fourth and even fifth waves are now throwing havoc in several countries.

Luckily, it became apparent recently that the Omicron variant is a mild one. Based on these findings, epidemiologists are saying that the virus may not reach a 'Herd Immunity' soon.

The significance of this conclusion is that if the virus will continue to spread in the world, it may become endemic[12]) - a risk that always lurks...

Professor Hyman, an epidemiologist and expert in infectious diseases and who had been a member of the epidemiological service of the CDC and a senior scientist in the WHO, said that the wide distribution of the Omicron variant raises the probability that it will have a permanent existence in most parts of the world!

According to Hyman, future outbreaks will be smaller than those which affected India and Brazil, because as time goes on, more people become infected and develop a certain immunity or become actively immunized. This is a natural development in infectious diseases in Humans (for example as in Tuberculosis and HIV)."

The vaccines were developed in record time, but their distribution in the globe proceeds slowly and in an un-

---

[12] *Endemic - In epidemiology, an infection is said to be endemic in a population when that infection is constantly maintained at a baseline level in a geographic area without external inputs.*

equitable manner. Rich countries amass vaccines while poor countries struggle with logistic problems in the distribution of those vaccines that they manage to obtain, in many countries the populations refuse to get vaccinated. Only a few countries managed to vaccinate, at least partially, about 70% of their citizens. Less than 10% of the immense population of India had been vaccinated at least partially.

In Africa, the number is less than 1%. Only a small number of countries in Africa, mostly Island countries, managed to keep the virus under control and will continue to do that as soon as they will succeed to immunize enough people.

In summary, our work is cut for us, and I hope that we will succeed!"

Here Jerry finished his talk and said: "That is all folks! I shall not answer any questions right now, because I think that our boss wants to let Josh start his presentation. I shall answer your questions after Josh's exposition. Feel free to approach me then!" Jerry went to his seat, followed by his colleagues' applause.

But Richard then addressed Josh and said: "Josh, I shall let you shine and impress your new colleagues with your knowledge on COVID-19's life cycle somewhat later. I Promise you that it will be soon! However, right now I am eager for us to start our work with our molecular biologists. We wasted 4 weeks until we were fully equipped and immunized, and now I am eager to start. Some of our competitors are probably already quite ahead of us. We need, as I described in my battle plan, to start a genetic modification plan of spike so that we shall be able to weaken the corona and remove its poison fangs. Therefore, please describe to all our colleagues all you know on the target of our work, namely the **spike!**

Chapter 1/6

The spike and its menacing juggling

Obeying Richard's request, Josh went to the screen in the front of the "class" and started his lecture on the spike.

"Dear colleagues, Coronaviruses are large, roughly spherical particles with unique surface projections that are called **"spikes."** According to the Linnaean classification system in Biology, because of their conservation of their "core replicase," Coronaviruses belong to the Coronavirideae family and to the order of Nidovirales, as Jerry had already taught us. This family includes the Severe Acute Respiratory Syndrome (SARS) virus (SARS-Cov), Middle East Respiratory Syndrome (MERS) virus (MERS-Cov) and SARS-CoV-2, the causative agent of the COVID-19 plague.

The functions that direct coronavirus' RNA synthesis and processing reside in nonstructural polyprotein (comprising of **nsp** 1 to **nsp** 16). These 16 proteins are cleavage products of a large replicase polyprotein translated directly from the infecting coronavirus genome.

The Coronaviridaeae viruses have polycistronic RNA genomes with several domains. Polycistronic RNA is an RNA that encodes (translates) several non-structural proteins (the **nsp1** to **nsp** 16 that I mentioned a few seconds ago) that follow one after the other. It consists of a leader sequence that precedes the first gene involved in mRNA capping (**nsp14**[13]) and **nsp16**) and fidelity control (**nsp** 14). Several smaller subunits in the mRNA (**nsp** 7-**nsp** 10) act as crucial cofactors of these nsp proteins. The Coronavirus' genomes with the size of ~26-32 kilo bases are the largest RNA genomes known to date. A considerable progress has now been made regarding their structural and functional properties. The Coronavirus' "replicase" function in the mRNA includes the proteins of the RNA polymerase (**nsp**12) and helicase (**nsp** 13). However, they also contain number of rare or even unique domains. The viral mRNA also produces 4 structural proteins (**sp**) and among these proteins we find the terrible SPIKE that is so important to our work, and that Richard asked me to describe to you:

Before the start of infection, he SPIKE protein is made of 5 units that are loosely aggregated into a spike that has a **stalk** and a **cap**. The stalk is inserted into the outer coat of the virus. When the cap touches the cell that is about to be infected, spike protein separate. There are three identical proteins of the type S1 and two identical proteins of the type S2.

The S1 Spike proteins attach during infection to a cellular receptor that is called ACE2, while the S2 proteins **fuse** at the same time with the host cell's

---

[13] *NSP -Non- structural proteins*

outer membrane and introduce the "nucleus" of the virus – its viral mRNA plus protein (**nucleoprotein**) into infected cell.

The COVID-19's spike proteins, when they are still aggregated, contain an insertion of a small sequence of four amino acids that are also present in the virulent zoonotic severe acute respiratory syndrome (SARS) virus that caused the pandemic of 2003. The amino acids that the peculiar insertion coded for, are arginine, arginine, alanine, and arginine. Their presence, so Decroly from the French Aix-Marseille University and his colleagues observed, may heighten the "pathogenicity" — that is, the god-awfulness — of the COVID-19 disease. This sequence of the 4 amino acids is easy to remember because it is like a roar: "R-R-A-R." (these are the letter-code that translates into the amino acids described above (arginine, arginine, alanine, and arginine). These four amino acids produce a cleavage site. This cleavage site is sensitive to a protease enzyme called Furin (an enzyme that is highly prevalent in the human body). The Furin cleavage site confers on the 5 spike proteins (three S1 and two S2) a form that looks like a "lobster's claw."

The cleavage site is in a boundary between the two types of subunits of the spike protein: the S1 subunits and S2 subunits. The French investigators said that when the COVID-19's spike senses Furin, it "shudders", chemically speaking, and the enzyme separates the loosely packed S1 and S2, that make up the spike. Here josh screened the figure of the spike with the" lobster's claw":

Lobster's claw

↓

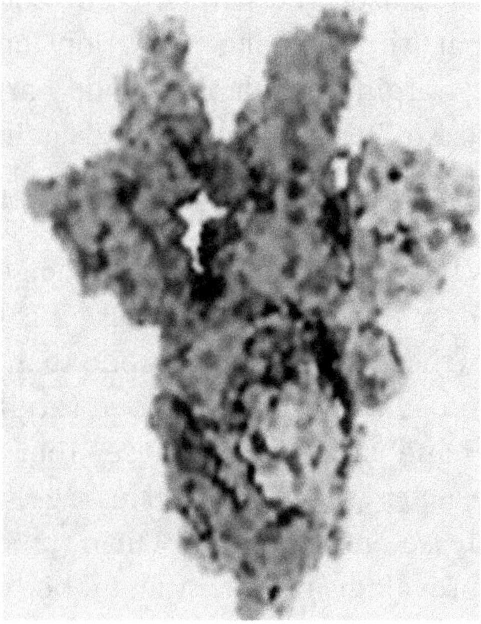

The net structural consequence of the insertion of the Furin cleavage site into the SARS-CoV-2 spike is that its S1 and S2 subunits will still be bonded together even if the Furin cleavage site is opened by the Furin protease. Let me repeat this crucial point: the COVID-19 uses its spike proteins (S1 and S2) to attach to the cellular receptor on the cell wall and to mediate viral entry into host cells by fusion.

For the Covs strains (other than COVID-19), that is the SARS and the MERS strains, there are a variety of proteases in addition to the Furin that are capable of priming and triggering the cleavage site in the spikes. These are proteases at the plasma membrane or endosomal membrane. Among them, the best known is the transmembrane-bound protease TMPRSS2. However, TMPRSS2's expression is limited to epithelial cell lines.

Here Josh cited a section from a paper by Veesler and colleagues from Seattle: "The spike is the **business part** as far as viral entry is concerned," Veesler explained. "It is in charge not only of attachment to the host cell surface, but also of fusing the viral and host cell membranes together to allow the infection to start. The spike is also the main target of neutralizing antibodies, so it is important for vaccine and therapeutic design."

Josh continued: "One finding in Vessler's recent research was that neutralizing antibodies that inhibit the cellular fusion into cells, are elicited by vaccination with the current RNA vaccines. As every conversant person in the world knows, the outer membrane of the COVID-19 virions has a crown-like appearance, because of its decoration with the glycoprotein spikes. The virion is surrounded by a membrane and an envelope that are attached together. These 2 membranes are speared (pierced) by the spikes. "Previous studies, and new ones, suggested that a spike proteins' adaptation caused a high affinity for human ACE2 receptor and may be related to the severity of the COVID-19's pandemic."

Here Josh projected a figure of the COVID virion. And said: "The figure shows the envelope-plus-membrane and the spikes stuck into it. It also contained the viral RNA which is mingled with nucleoproteins "beads." Then he continued his with his spike discourse:

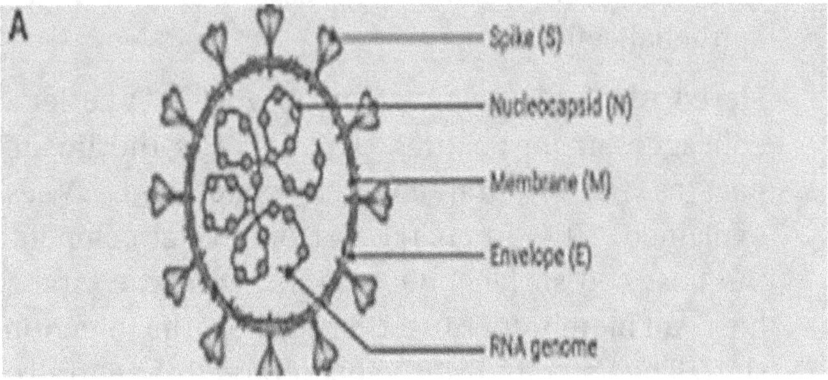

"The crown (**corona** in Latin) gives the COVID-19 its family name. The combined viral RNA plus the protein beads **nucleoprotein**).

The two subunits remain noncovalently linked on the viral surface, until the attachment onto the host cell membrane. In a functionally active state, three S1s are attached to two S2 subunits.

Now I want to compare a figure that depicts, a closed spike, an open spike, and a spike with the Furin cleavage site that additional studies by more groups showed that it enhances the ability of COVID-19 to infect.

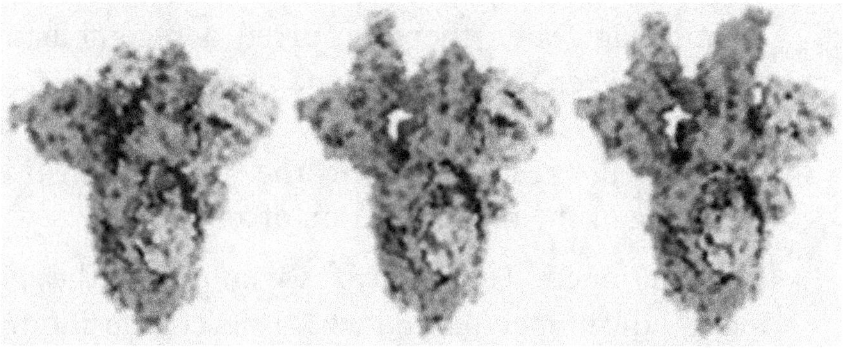

Closed S proteins Open S proteins Open GS14 mutant

A Professor by the name of Fang Chi-tai of the National Taiwan University, also reacted on this matter of the cleavage site and the possibility that the COVID-19 became zoonotic not by Nature, but by human hands. As I already described to you, it was found that the anomalous Furin cleavage site in the spike is made by the addition of 4 amino acids with the symbols of R-R-A-R that stand for arginine, arginine, alanine, and arginine.

Fang Chi Tai said that the virus was unlikely to have four amino acids added all at once. Natural mutations are smaller and more haphazard. Therefore, it is quite possible that the amino acids were added to the COVID-19 in the high security lab of the Wuhan institute of virology's by humans!"

Josh continued: "This statement of Fang Chi Tai opened a controversy because there is also an opposing opinion on the origin of COVID-19: This opinion states that as with several other coronaviruses, the COVID-19 virus probably originated in a species of a bat which infected a mammalian. Then there occurred a recombination event between the bat virus and the animal virus, and the COVID-19 virus became zoonotic. However, there is no real proof for the Chinese institute pottering or the recombination of a bat virus."

Josh continued: "How is it that we know how the spike looks, how it operates and what is its composition?

Very recent innovations in imaging techniques enabled researchers to peer closely at the virus' spike. The scientists managed to create a model of the spike, right down to the atoms and are beginning to unravel its secrets. The imaging technic used is called FRET and I shall describe in a moment. At present, I shall just say that the region of the viral mRNA that translates the Spike is in the last third of the mRNA. This third part of starts with the open reading frame of 1b(ORF1b) codes, The spike is coded together with additional structural proteins that go to construct the virion. These are the Envelope (E), Membrane (M) and nucleoprotein (N)]."

Chapter 1/7

The various FRET conformations of the spike

Josh continued: "Now I want to describe to you how the FRET technic works and to discuss the various conformations in which the spike can exist. This discussion will also show how the conformations that the spike can present affect, the attachment of the spike's S2 proteins to the cell membrane.

FRET stands for "Single-molecule Förster Resonance Energy Transfer method (FRET)." This method has revealed how the different SARS-CoV-2 spike proteins are interconnected and the various conformations that they present.

In FRET, energy is transferred between two green Laser Fluorescent light-sensitive molecules. Since the efficiency of energy-transfer between 2 molecules is related to the distance between them in the FRET, this efficiency of energy-transfer is used to determine the distance between two parts of a molecule to which the light-sensitive molecules are attached. The FRET studies have revealed that in one conformation, all the RBDs (Receptor-Binding Domains[14]) of the S1 are oriented **downwards,** so that these domains are

---

[14] *Receptor binding domains - This loop dominant RBD consisting of 273 amino acids, is only part of the whole S protein, extending from residue 319 to 591. This region is key to the protein-receptor binding.*

inaccessible for binding to the infected cell. A second conformation is, where one or two RBDs are oriented **upwards,** and a third conformation in which all the RBDs of the spike are oriented **upwards** - all the receptor binding domains are accessible for attachment to the infected cell.

The researchers found low FRET efficiency (about 0.1), intermediate FRET efficiency (about 0.3 and 0.5), and high FRET efficiency (about 0.8). They say that these efficiencies correspond to at least four different conformations of the spike protein. The conformation with the intermediate FRET efficiency was the most abundant, based on counting several hundred FRET tracings. The authors said that this intermediate conformation corresponds to all the binding regions pointing **downward**, toward the intended infected cell surface. They found that a disulfide bridge between two amino acids stabilizes the **downward** orientation of the spike protein.

When they added isolated cellular ACE2 receptor proteins (angiotensin) that, as you remember, attaches to the binding regions of the spike, they found that the previously low FRET state was now more abundant, suggesting that all the RBDs, when bound to the isolated human receptors, are oriented in the **upward** direction, (away from the virus-surface).

The spike proteins were in equilibrium between the different conformations at physiological pH and room temperature. When the conformations changed, there was a specific order in which they transitioned; first from the **low** to the **intermediate** efficiency state, and then from the **intermediate** to the **high** efficiency state. Thus, there is a specific sequence of activating structural transitions in the SARS-CoV-2 spike protein: The RBD-**down** conformation changes to the RBD-**up** conformation, via at least one intermediate conformation which is activated by the ACE2 enzymatic cellular receptor.

Next, the FRET team analyzed what happens to the spike proteins' conformations when spike antibodies bind to them. Using antibodies isolated from the plasma of convalescent patients, which attached to the spike proteins, they found that the spike proteins were now in the **up** conformation. This was like the same orientation obtained using the isolated ACE2 receptor. In summary: the results suggest that the SARS-CoV-2 virus may be neutralized by diverse ways. In both instances, a stabilizing of the spike proteins in the **down** conformation, prevented a binding of the virus to the host cell."

Then Jerry added: "A few minutes ago, I described to you a peculiar insertion that adds virulence to the COVID-19. I want to elaborate on it some more. Recently, a dangerous mutation called G614 came into play in **all** variants. This mutation yields a wider open spike. The opening here looks like a "lobster claw." I have already described it to you before, but I neglected to tell you that **it is universally present in all current mutations!!!"**

With this statement, Josh finished his spike's lecture, went back to his seat and he received the applause of his colleagues and of Richard.

Chapter 1/8

Josh describes the CRISPR/Cas9 technic

Now Richard addressed Josh again and said: "Josh, now I want you to continue with your expositions and enlighten the virologists in our group on the CRISPR/Cas9 technic for editing nucleic acids.

Our molecular biologists used the technic many times, as they indicated in their application forms. Therefore, they are familiar with the technic. As for you, Josh, I sent you to Doudna's laboratory to learn all you can on the CRISPR/Cas9 editing technic. My colleagues, I am sure that you know that Professor Doudna was one of two women scientists who received a Nobel prize in the past year for the development of the technic. Since we are going to use this technic, in our modification experiments, I you to teach us this technic to the best of your ability."

Josh acceded to his boss' request and continued:

"Dear colleagues! Here goes: The CRISPR/Cas9 technique is just one of several gene-editing tools. However, many molecular biologists and geneticists favor this technique because of its high degree of flexibility and accuracy in cutting and pasting additional DNA. One of the reasons for its popularity, is that it makes it possible to carry out genetic engineering on an unprecedented scale and at an exceptionally low cost. It differs from previous genetic engineering techniques in that it allows the introduction or removal of more than one gene at a time. This makes it possible to manipulate, very quickly, many different genes in plant or animal cells thus reducing the process from taking several years, to a matter of weeks. It is also different in that it is not species-specific, so it can be used on organisms previously resistant to genetic engineering.

The technique is already being explored for a wide number of applications in fields ranging from agriculture to human health. In agriculture it can help in the design of new grains, roots, and fruits.

Within the context of Health, it could pave the way to the development of new treatments for rare metabolic disorders and genetic diseases, ranging from hemophilia to cystic fibrosis and to Huntingdon's disease. It is also now being utilized in the creation of transgenic animals to produce organs for transplantations into human patients. Several start-up companies exploit the technology commercially and large pharmaceutical companies are also exploring its use for drug-discovery and development purposes.

As Richard told us, the importance of the CRISPR/Cas9 was recognized with the awarding of the Nobel Prize in Chemistry to Jennifer Doudna and Emmanuel Charpentier in October 2020. But what was missed in the awarding notices of the Prize is the significant role that many others, mostly Virginijus Siksnys, a Lithuanian biochemist who also played a role in helping to bring about the development of gene-editing and worked on restriction (cutting) enzymes.

Here is a brief description of how the technic gradually evolved: In 1987 a Japanese team of scientists at Osaka University noticed a strange pattern of DNA sequences in a gene belonging to the well-known Escherichia coli bacterium. That gene had five short repeating segments of DNA separated by short non-repeating 'spacer' DNA sequences. All five repeating segments had identical sequences composed of 29 DNA bases. By contrast, each of the 'spacer' sequences had its own unique sequence, composed of thirty-two bases.

Microbiologists had never seen such a pattern before. By the end of the 1990s, however, the Osaka team had begun to discover, with the aid of new improvements to DNA sequencing, that this pattern was prevalent in many different microbe species.

So common was the pattern that it was given its own name: 'Clustered Regularly Inter-Spaced Short Palindromic repeats' – CRISPR for short. The term was coined by a team of Dutch scientists led by Rudd Jansen at Utrecht University, in 2002, who in the same year discovered that another set of sequences always accompanied the CRISPR sequence. They dubbed this second set of sequences 'Cas/ genes,' an abbreviation for CRISPR-associated genes. The Cas genes appeared to code for enzymes that cut DNA. By 2005 three scientific teams had independently worked out that the 'spacer' sequences between the CRISP sequences, shared similarities with the DNA of viruses of bacteria (bacteriophages) and hypothesized that it could be a tool in the defense mechanism of bacteria against these viruses.

Knowledge about how the CRISPR/Cas 9 system worked was opened by some experiments conducted in 2007 by scientists at Danisco, a Danish food manufacturer later acquired by DuPont. The team infected a milk-fermenting microbe, Streptococcus thermophilus, with two bacteriophage strains. Many of these bacteria were killed by the bacteriophages, but some bacteria survived and went on to produce offspring resistant to the bacteriophages. On further investigation, the resistant microbes were inserting DNA fragments from the bacteriophages into their 'spacer' sequences[15], and that they have lost the resistance whenever the new 'spacer' sequences were cut out.

In 2008 Eugene Koonin and colleagues at the National Center for Biotechnology Information in Bethesda, Maryland, demonstrated for the first time how the CRISPR/Cas 9 mechanism worked: Whenever bacteria confront an invader, such as a bacteriophage, they copy and incorporate a DNA segment from the bacteriophage into their genome as 'spacers' between the short DNA repeats in CRISPR. The segments in

---

[15] *Spacer sequences- Spacer DNA sequence are regions of non-coding DNA between genes. The terms intergenic spacer (IGS) or non-transcribed spacer (NGS) are used particularly for the spacer DNA between the many tandemly repeated DNA copies.*

the 'spacers' provide a template for the bacteria's RNA molecules to recognize any future DNA of an incoming bacteriophage and guide the Cas/9 enzyme to cut it up, thereby disabling the bacteriophages.

As Richard already mentioned, four years later, a small team of scientists led by Jennifer Doudna, University California, Berkeley, and Emmanuelle Charpentier, University of Umea, (a Swedish University), published a paper showing how to harness the natural CRISPR-/Cas 9 system as a tool to cut any DNA strand in a test tube. Shortly before, Virginijus Siksnys at Vilnius University, independently submitted a paper to "Cell," elucidating the potential of CRISPR/Cas9 for gene editing in a paper. The editor of "Cell" rejected the manuscript without sending it out for review. Siksnys eventually had his article published in the Proceedings of the National Academic of Sciences. A year later, in January 2013, several researchers at different laboratories published papers within a few weeks of each other demonstrating how the CRISPR/Cas 9 system could be used to edit genomes in human cells. This included teams led by Doudna, Feng Zhang at MIT-Harvard Broad Institute, and George Church at Harvard Medical School.

Several changes are now underway to improve the accuracy and efficiency of the CRISPR/Cas 9 technic. A key breakthrough has been the development of new Cas 9 fusion proteins to act as base (nucleoside) editors.

The fusion proteins make it possible to convert cytosine to uracil without cutting DNA. Uracil is subsequently transformed into thymine through DNA replication or repair. The first "base editors" were generated in 2016 by Alexis Komor and colleagues in the laboratory of David Liu at Harvard University.

The first application of the CRISPR/Cas 9 system was first exploited by Danisco in 2008 as I already described to you. The company used it to improve the immunity of bacterial cultures against bacteriophages. Many food manufacturers now use the technology to produce cheese and yoghurt. Since then, the technology has been used to delete, insert, and modify DNA in human cells and other animal cells grown in petri dishes. Scientists are also using it to create transgenic animals such as mice, rats, pigs, and primates.

Between 2014 and 2015 scientists reported the successful use of CRISPR/Cas 9 in mice to eliminate muscular dystrophy, to cure rare liver disease, and to make human cells immune to HIV. It is also being Investigated in conjunction with stem cells[16]) to provide human organs from transgenic pigs. Such

---

[16] *Stem cells- Stem cells are the body's raw materials—cells from which all other cells with specialized functions are generated. Under the right conditions in the body or a laboratory, stem cells divide to form more cells called daughter cells. These daughter cells either become new stem cells (self-renewal) or become specialized cells (differentiation) with a more specific function such as blood cells, brain cells, heart muscle cells or bone cells. No other cell in the body has the natural ability to generate new cell types.*

work is directed towards helping solve some of the shortage of human organs for transplant operations and overcome some of the side-effects caused by organ transplantation such as graft-versus host disease) where the transplanted organ induces immunity against the host."

Now, I will describe the important points of the CRISPR:

Scientists start with a fragment of synthesized RNA that contains the gene, or fragment, or base that must be altered/repaired. That is a molecule that can read the genetic information in DNA. The RNA finds the spot in the nucleus of a cell where some editing activity should take place. This guide RNA directs the Cas9 to the precise spot in the DNA where a cut is called for. Cas9 then locks onto the double-stranded DNA and unzips it.

This allows the above guide RNA to pair up with the target region of the DNA. Cas 9 snips the DNA at this spot. This creates a break in both strands of the DNA molecule. The cell, sensing a problem, repairs the break. Fixing the break might disable a gene (the easiest thing to do). Alternatively, this repair might fix a mistake or even insert a new gene or a base (a much more complicated process).

Cells usually repair a break in their DNA by gluing the loose ends back together. That is a sloppy process. It often results in a mistake that disables some gene. That may not sound useful — but sometimes it is.

Scientists cut DNA with CRISPR/Cas 9 to make gene changes, or mutations. By comparing cells with and without the mutation, scientists can sometimes figure out what a protein's normal role is. Or a new mutation may help them understand genetic diseases. CRISPR/Cas 9 also can be useful in human cells by disabling certain genes — ones, for instance, which play a role in inherited diseases.

The original Cas 9 is like a Swiss army knife with only one application. But this knife which have been dulled, in the updated version has attached to it other proteins and chemicals. That has transformed that knife into a multifunctional tool.

CRISPR/Cas 9 and related tools can now be used in new ways, such as changing a single nucleotide base — a single letter in the genetic code or adding a fluorescent protein to tag a spot in the DNA that scientists want to track. Scientists also can use this genetic cut-and-paste technology to turn genes on or off.

With this description of how CRISPR works, Josh completed his presentation and sat down, followed by the applause of his colleagues, also including those of the boss.

Chapter 1/9

Jane describes the "Prime editing" of Nucleic Acids: RNA and DNA

Richard then addressed his colleagues: "Hi team, Josh taught a lot about the CRISPR and its theory. Now I need someone who is a bit more experienced to teach us more. This is because the original CRISPR is evolving very rapidly by several scientists. Josh, I apologize for wishing to learn more! I have worked once with the CRISPR/Cas9, but I am far from being an expert. Therefore, I recruited two excellent molecular biologists –Jane and Jim --to help us. There is now an important breakthrough in the method that I read about. I want to ask Jane and Jim to teach use this latest advance. I asked Jane and Jim, and both told me that they have already worked with it."

Then, addressing the team's molecular biologist she said: "Dear friends, could you share with us your newest knowledge on the CRISPR?"

Both scientists enthusiastically agreed. They conferred for a minute, and then Jane said: "by a unanimous decision it was decided that I shall be the tutor this time."

Jane went to the front of the" class" and immediately started:

“The newest wrinkle in the method. “Prime editing,” was developed by Anzalone and Liu and colleagues from the Broad Institute of MIT and Harvard. It uses a longer-than-usual guide RNA called the prime editor, a guide RNA (pegRNA) and a fusion protein consisting of Cas9 H840A Nickase enzyme fused to a specially engineered reverse transcriptase enzyme. Anzalone and Liu and their colleagues tested whether single guide RNA (sgRNA) could be extended to include extra bases. Some of these extra bases would serve as a template for synthesis of a new DNA sequence, and others would bind to the DNA strand opposite from the normal sgRNA binding site.

They aimed to use that area of the DNA as a primer for reverse transcriptase. They found that their long RNA, called pegRNA, was able to guide the Cas9 enzyme to its correct target and trigger genome editing. The scientists also introduced another guide RNA in addition to the pegRNA. This additional guide RNA was sgRNA that directed the Cas9 H840A Nickase to nick the genomic DNA at a nearby site but on the opposite strand as the original nick. The reason for doing this was a concern that good editing of one strand would be removed due to a mismatch between the edited and non-edited strands. By introducing a nick on the non-edited strand, the scientists reasoned that the cell’s natural repair systems might remove the original sequence and replace it with the edited sequence in the parallel strand. Indeed, Anzalone et al. found that this worked well. It even worked better when a second sgRNA sequence could be designed to match the newly edited sequence introduced by the pegRNA. Anzalone et al. tested the ability of their method of prime editing to insert and then to correct several known pathogenic mutations in various human cell lines that bore the pathogenic mutations.

How is it that Prime Editing does not cause breaks in the double stranded DNA genome, yet still manages to edit the genome? This is where the genius of Prime Editing comes into play. PegRNA uses its Cas9 type enzyme Nickase (the traditional Cas9 enzyme). The Nickase enzyme is specially fused engineered reverse transcriptase enzyme as I already described. What the Nickase does is it cuts only one strand the DNA of its two strands (like the traditional Cas9 does).The correcting long single stranded RNA is joined into the site of the cut. The reverse transcriptase then completes the synthesis of the complementary strand. Jane finished her lesson with the customary applause…

Chapter 1/10

Jerry describes the life cycle of COVID-19

After the completion of Jane's lesson, Richard, as an orchestra conductor, Invited Jerry to talk about COVID-19'S synthesis of proteins and RNA. To do that, Jerry first screened on the whiteboard chart published by a company called "Genetic Education Inc." While doing this he said: "I selected this chart out of quite a few other ones in the Wikipedia and it will help you to follow on whatever I am speaking. It is a simple, but the informative chart and I to repeatedly during my discourse!

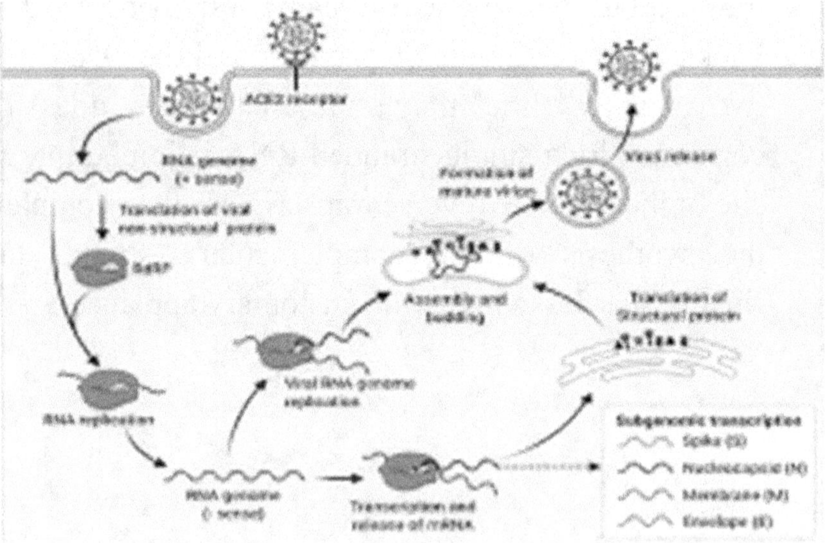

COVID-19'S life cycle

While screening the scheme, Josh said: “Dear colleagues and boss-colleague! In a sense, my dissertation is redundant. The “Genetic Education Inc.’s scheme that I projected before you describe everything in the life cycle of the COVID-19.

Still, let me describe to you the life cycle of the virus, how it infects a cell, and translates its protein and transcribes new virions in the infected host only.

The SARS-Cov-2 was named first as nCoV-2019 and now is mostly called COVID -19, a name conceived by the WHO.

The epicenter[17]) of COVID-19 outbreak was in the city of Wuhan in Hubei Province of central China and its Huanan seafood wholesale market. The COVID-19 is a type of retrovirus pseudo type (it is not true retrovirus, but it has features that are reminiscent of the replication of the HIV virus). It infects especially mammals and birds. However, the signs and symptoms of the infection are more serious in humans.

TheCOVID-19virus belongs systematically to the Nidovirales order and the. Positive-strand RNA genome and a rigid envelope are unique characteristics of the viruses of this family.

Electron microscope studies reveal that the virions of SARS-CoV-2 are spherical shaped, 125nm in

---

[17] *Epicenter of the outbreak– The focus of infection – where the infection started.*

diameter, and have spike protein on its surface. The MERS-CoV and SARS-CoV from the same systematic family AS covid-19, were transmitted to humans from camels and civet cats, respectively. Both these strains are not so lethal, unlike SARS-CoV-2 (COVID-19) which evolved recently after an infection from bats to an intermediate animal – a Pangolin anteater.

Jerry said: "Let us first concentrate first on the COVID-19's proteins. The virus contains genetic information (mRNA) for the synthesis of three classes of proteins:

1) Structural proteins (**sp**) that are assembled into the COVID virion.
2) Non- structural proteins (**nsp**) that participate in the viral replication and are not assembled into the virion.
3) Accessory proteins whose role is to inhibit the body's natural defenses.

COVID-19 contains a single-stranded (positive-sense) RNA associated with a nucleoprotein within a capsid comprised of matrix protein. The COVID 19'sRNA contains at least six ORFs (Open Reading Frames). The first ORF (1a and 1b) encodes a large polyprotein that is cleaved into nonstructural proteins (**nsp**). All the structural (four in number) and accessory proteins are translated from the ORFs 10 and 11 which are on the one-third of the end of the genome near the 3'-terminus. These four structural proteins are the Spike, Membrane, Nucleocapsid and Envelope proteins. This part of viral mRNA also encodes eight SARS-CoV-specific accessory proteins (3a,3b,6, 7a, 7b, 8a, 8b and 9b).

The four structural proteins are as follows:

1. The **notorious criminal spike** (S),

2. The Nucleocapsid proteins that like beads on a string, attach to the internal mRNA in the very center of the virion. Because of their binding to the mRNA, they stabilize it. nucleocapsids(N),

3. The membrane proteins that are designated (M), and:

4. Envelope proteins that are designated as (E). Together with the M proteins, the envelope proteins produce a double capsule around the stabilized mRNA.

My esteemed colleagues, please observe now again the scheme of the infection cycle and see these proteins.

But now, let us talk about the viral mRNA:

The mRNA is a positive-sense genomic RNA which, when it is freed from the virus capsule after the attachment and fusion of the spike's S1 and S2 proteins, it becomes the template to produce the structural and non-structural proteins. This is done by translation[18])_together with ribosomes and tRNAs. The mRNA also becomes the template for the multiplication by transcription[19]) of new mRNA for the new progeny viruses.

RNA translation occurs inside the endoplasmic reticulum (ER). The viral structural proteins move along the secretory pathway into the Golgi intermediate compartment. There, the M proteins direct the protein-protein interactions required for the assembly of the viral RNA (after its binding to the nucleocapsid). This assembly creates complete virions for further infections of new cells.

The viral RNA (with its capsid proteins) has a helical symmetry. It is enclosed in an envelope made of a lipid bilayer (from the infected cell), and the various structural proteins: The Nucleoproteins (N), the membrane proteins (M), and envelope proteins (E) protect the virus when its "streams" inside the body. The spike (S) is also included in the protection of the RNA, because it is glycosylated.

The ratio of the structural proteins-E:S:M in the lipid bilayer-is1:20:300. The E and M proteins are the structural proteins that, combined with the lipid bilayer of the infected cell, shape the viral envelope,

---

[18] *Translation-Translation is a process by which polypeptides (proteins) are synthesized from mRNA transcript. During this process, tRNA acts as a carrier by bringing with it specific amino acids to the ribosomes to produce a growing protein..*

[19] *Transcription -Transcription is the process of making an RNA copy of a gene sequence. This copy, called a messenger RN(mRNA)molecule, leaves the cell nucleus, and enters the cytoplasm, where it directs the synthesis of the protein, which it encodes.*

and maintain its size. As Josh already told us, the spikes are inserted (pierced) into the assembled envelope. The thickness of the envelope is 85 nm. In electron micrographs, the assembled envelope of the virus appears as a distinct pair of electron dense circles (electron dense means that they are opaque to the electron beam used to scan the virus particle).

The M protein is the main structural protein of the envelope that provides the overall shape. It consists of 218 to 263 amino acid residues and forms a layer 7.8 nm thick. It has three domains[20]), a short N-terminal ectodomain, a triple-spanning transmembrane domain, and a C-terminal end domain. The C-terminal domain forms a matrix-like lattice that adds to the extra thickness of the envelope.

The M protein is crucial during the assembly, budding, envelope formation, and pathogenesis stages of the virus lifecycle.

The E proteins are minor structural proteins. There are only about twenty copies of the E protein molecule in a coronavirus particle. They are 8.4 to 12 kilo-Dalton in size and are composed of 76 to 109 amino acids. They are integral proteins (i.e., embedded in the lipid layer) and have two domains (transmembrane domain and an extra membrane C-terminal domain). They are fully α-helical, with a

---

[20] *The term domain in biochemistry and molecular virology is used to refer to a part of a protein that has a conserved structure and function, is similar between related proteins, and can exist or function on its own if it was separated from the rest of the protein.*

single α-helical transmembrane domain, and form pentameric (five-molecular) ion channels in the lipid bilayer. They are responsible for virion assembly, intracellular transport, and acquisition of form by the virions.

The M and E proteins are primarily involved in virus assembly.

Inside the envelope, there is the nucleocapsid, which is formed from multiple copies of the nucleocapsid (N) protein. The N protein is a phosphoprotein of 43 to 50 kilo-Dalton in size and is divided into three conserved domains. Their domains 1 and 2, are typically rich in Arginines and Lysines. The nucleoproteins have a net negative charge due to excess of acidic over basic amino acid residues.

As I already told you, the viral genome is a positive-sense, single-stranded RNA. Its size is 26.4 to 31.7 kilobases[21]) and it is one of the largest among RNA viruses. The infecting plus sense mRNA immediately acts upon its uncoating as a messenger RNA. After translation it is replicated (transcribed) by the RNA dependent RNA polymerase (RdRP).

Each of the two mRNA regions has a 5′ methylated cap as a starting point, anda3′polyadenylatedtail as the ending point of the translation. This allows them to act as the messenger RNAs that they are. Some of the nonstructural proteins form a **replication**

---

21 *A Kilobase is one thousand bases. Expresses the lengths of nucleic acid molecules*

complex that contains the RNA-dependent RNA polymerase (RdRP). This enzyme synthesizes a full-length minus sense strand of RNA which is the template for the synthesis of the complementary+ sense RNA that is packaged into the new virions as I described to you a few minutes ago.

The newly synthesized structural and accessory proteins are then transferred from the ER through the Golgi apparatus, after which new virions assemble in budding Golgi vesicles. Finally, the mature SARS-CoV-2 virions are exocytosed[22]) and released from the host cell into the surrounding environment to repeat the infection cycle.

I just want to add that the viral RNA is folded and stabilized by the nucleocapsid proteins that attach to it like pearls on a string.

Jerry finished his discourse and sat down, but not without receiving Accolades from his teammates which also included Richard.

---

[22] *Exocytosis-Exocytosis is the natural process of transporting molecules (including viruses) from within a cell to the outside space. In this process, the vesicles containing the fluid enclosed by a lipid bilayer fuse with the plasma membrane to release their contents outside the cell.*

Chapter 1/11

Armageddon, the Götterdämmerung, the Tempest and Ragnarök, "and the rats will inherit the earth!"

Then Richard said: "Dear colleagues: As I have told you before, there are several groups of scientists who work on the same project that we intend to pursue. We lost a whole month getting ready to start and I know that we must work very quickly and hard to regain the time that we lost and pursue our competitors.

Now we need to move quickly, but with great inventiveness, to plan our attack on the spike! But first, I want to summarize what we know on the various dangerous mutations of the spike relative to the Wuhan variant and its innocent and non-zoonotic RaTG13 that Shi Zhengli, "bat-woman" culled from the droppings of a bat in the Yunnan province. The professor added: now I am screening a slide of the various variants and their spike mutations:

List of the torture trail of Covid variants

Variant	Mutation	Infectivity
Wuhan	D614G	Globally dominant mutation
Cluster "5'	D614G, Y453F	More infectious than the Wuhan variant
British	D614G	More infectious than the Wuhan variant
Brazilian	D614G, E484K	More infectious than the Wuhan variant
Indian (Delta)	D614G, L452R, E484Q	Very infectious
South African	D614G, K417N, E484K,N501Y	Highly infectious
Omicron	D614G	Extremely infectious
BA2	D614G	Extremely infectious

Dear readers! Here we are approaching the danger point of the reckless modification of the COVID-19. **(Read it and fear!)**

The professor continued: The Spike protein (S) is a string of 1,273 amino acids; in the original form from Wuhan the 614th of these amino acids has the chemical symbol "D" (aspartic acid), while in the mutated form, the 614th amino acid is abbreviated to "G" (glycine). So D614G) is short for "having a Spike protein with aspartic acid at position 614 of the spike mutated to glycine." G614 is already a dangerous mutation. As Josh has already told us, this mutation yields a wider open spike that looks like a "lobster claw" and has already been described by Josh.

However, the G614 did not stop its mischief just there. It showed a great propensity to easily mutate back to its original harmless variant D614. From there it was just an easy step to become the D614G mutation with an extremely high infectivity rate to-date. This is the mutant that accounts for its rapid rise to the dominant position in all regions where it has emerged. D614G is one candidate that we are going to modify.

The second candidate that we are going to pick for modification is E484K with the amino acids glutamate (E) and lysine (K). The third candidate is the Indian variant L452R. This L452R mutation swaps out the leucine amino acid (L) for the arginine amino acid (R). As the virus replicates, it develops further mutations. Some mutations cause the spike to change shape by adding or deleting amino acids, which can affect the way it interacts with the human ACE2 receptor on the surface of many cells. It binds strongly to the ACE2. India has now a second variant side by side to the L452Rmutation. This is E484Q, whereby the glutamic acid (E) is replaced by glutamine (Q) at position 484. This is our fourth candidate for modification.

I know that I asked all of you to show inventiveness and to suggest modifications. However, as your boss, I want to suggest a modification that Jane and Jim will immediately start to modify. I think that all of you will agree with my choice of the first variant that I already chose. It is not the worst mutation, but it is going to be a test case for us to see if we can indeed modify COVID-19 variants.

Now, between us, when it will be your turn to suggest a modification of the RNA, you shall need to decide how to modify the mutant that you chose according to the following criteria:

a) To remove one amino acid.
b) To remove several amino acids in a string or in various places.
c) To exchange one amino acid for another.
d) To exchange several amino in a string or in several places.

As you can see, if we are going to enter a modification mode, we will have to make multiple choices. It is not like an examination with just four choices... At first, we shall use the capabilities of our molecular biologists Jane and Jim who are specialists in the operation of the various CRISPR technics for the editing of nucleic acids. They will apply the pegRNA editor which is the latest, and the best so far "wrinkle" in RNA editing. It uses a longer-than-usual guide RNA called the “prime editor,” a guide RNA (pegRNA) and a fusion protein consisting of Cas9 H840A Nickase enzyme fused to a specially engineered reverse transcriptase enzyme. In our very first exercise in editing, we shall Exchange in D614G Proline (Pro), instead of G (glycine). I do not expect this exchange to yield us a low infectivity modification unless by an extremely fortunate case. This is to learn the PegRNA editing technic.

Dear colleagues, do not worry. As I said Josh will teach you the Duodena CRISPR Cas technic, and either Jane or Jim will teach you the PegRNA technic.

How are we going to proceed with our modification?

I requested Dr. Shi Zhengli to send me the original non-zoonotic mutant - RaTG13. From the WHO I received the D614G mutant. To remind you - in this mutant, the 614th amino acid is abbreviated “G” (glycine); so D614G) is short for “having a Spike protein with aspartic acid at position 614 of the spike mutated to glycine.

Also, I asked the chairmen of Pfizer to send me have some of the lipid nanoparticles that the company used to coat their naked RNA vaccine. He sent me back ten pounds of their lipid nanoparticles. He also told me the inventor of the nanoparticles, Professor Weissman tested forty diverse types of delivery systems until he and he team, found their golden ticket: lipid nanoparticles. These “droplets of fat” coat the mRNA and allow it to successfully enter our cells and avoid being chewed up by cellular enzymes. Traditional vaccines are typically formulated with adjuvants that are designed to stimulate the immune response in their recipients. In what Weissman described as his lucky development, lipid nanoparticles happened to act also as an adjuvant that stimulated a specific type of "helper cell" that promotes antibody responses.

Pfizer says it uses four different lipids to produce the nanoparticles for the envelope in a "defined ratio."

One ingredient in the formulation of the Pfizer's vaccine is known. That is ALC-0315 which is the primary ingredient. That is because it is ionizable— it can be given a positive charge, and since the RNA has a negative one, they stick together.

The other lipids, one of which is the molecule of cholesterol, are liposomes. They are "helpers" that give structural integrity to the nanoparticles or stop them from clumping. During manufacturing, the RNA and the lipids are stirred into a bubbly mix.

We shall start by extracting the RNA of the two COVID-19 variants that I mentioned RNA with TRIzol) reagent and then we shall modify only the 2 RNAs with the PegRNA method.

In the next step we shall coat the two modified RNAs with the Nano particles lipid coat and infect a tissue-cultured hamster cell line with each of the two modified variants. The nanoparticle-l lipid-coated

RNA will act as a live virus and will infect the BHK cells, producing a new progeny virus and destroying the cell.

We will harvest the control (unmodified RaTG13 control virions) and the modified D614G (now D614G). Each of the types of the virions will be injected into four hamsters in our animal house and we shall observe the hamsters for infectivity! Here is a table that summarizes the steps that we will follow in our experimental training procedure. Here is a table that summarized our actions during the training exercise (the professor screened the table):

MODIFICATION PROCEDURE NUMBER 1

Variant for modification	RaTG13 (control)	D614G
Type of modification	none	Modify D614G to D614Pro (Pro – Proline)
Extracting solution	TRIzol	TRIzol
Type of CRISPR	none	PegRNA
Protective coat of the RNA	Lipid Nanoparticles	Lipid Nanoparticles
Cultured Cell line infected	BHK21 (baby hamster kidney cell line)	BHK21 (baby hamster kidney cell line)
Infection of four hamsters With the isolated virions	Infection	Infection
Daily observation of the proceeding d of infectivity	Observation and base sequencing of virus purified from the RNA-	Observation and base sequencing of the modifies virus

Dear Readers!

The team caried out the training experiment with Jane and Jim performing the pegRNA part. Now all that remained for the scientists to do is to wait patiently for the outcome of the experiment.

On the first, second and third day they had nothing to report, as they expected. On the morning of the fourth day, the scientists gathered to a brainstorming meeting in which they were supposed to decide on a "real" modification experiment. The professor started to speak when an urgent knocking on the door interrupted him, from second to second the knocking grew louder a more urgent. Josh went to open the door and in stumbled Jeff. The chief animal tender in their secured animal house. He looked distraught, coughed uncontrollably, and all the signs of elevated temperature.

The professor ran to Jeff and started to interrogate him. Interrupted by cough Jeff managed to whisper that he thinks that he got some bug. Upon further questioning he lisped that on the previous day, the four hamsters in the cage labelled "D614Pro" started to act maniacally and attacked each other. Jeff decided to put every hamster in a separate cage. Therefore, he grabbed one hamster and another hamster ran quickly along his arm and bit him in an area which was not covered by his protective glove...!

Jeff managed to stammer that he disinfected the small bite and thought nothing more of it. But, after a sleep interrupted by a nightmare, S woke up delirious and flushed and his wife demanded that he would talk to the professor and ask one of the professor's team to drive him to the ER in the closest hospital. The professor blanched, and so did some of his more astute of post-Docs. The entire world was swept by an extremely infective and lethal pandemic!!! Corpses littered the entire world rotting without any burial where they keeled. The professor went on print in one of the few remaining newspapers on the second day of the "Armageddon, the Gotterdammerung, the Tempest and Ragnarök," and admitted his sins. Then, on the same day he did not wait for the obvious outcome and blew a hole in his head....

Appendix: How did the SARS- Cov-2 come to infect humans? Who shall shoulder the blame?

The present appendix is intended to discuss the question of how the COVID-19 came to shake our world. Some of the points in this appendix have already discussed in the novelette till now and are repeated for the sake of clarity. Unfortunately, no real conclusion can come from this appendix. Still, I decided to bring it for the readers to let them form their own conclusions on the source of COVID-19:

In an article in the New York magazine "Intelligencer' Nicholson Baker, an American novelist and essayist. wrote: "The Chinese government said that the virus came to infect humans from seafood in the maritime market in Wuhan - a port in east-central China which is the capital of Hubei province. It is situated at the meeting of the Han and the Yangtze Rivers.

Following these announcements of the Chinese government, Doctor Li- Meng Yan, a scientist who conducted some of the earliest research on coronaviruses, claimed in a publicly open-access website that "COVID-19 could be "conveniently created" in a laboratory setting within six months."

Her claim was that the COVID-19 virus shows biological characteristics that are inconsistent with a naturally occurring, zoonotic virus. In her report, she described the genomic, structural, medical, and literature evidence, which, when considered together, strongly contradicts the "natural origin" theory. She insisted that the Wuhan variant comes from the lab in Wuhan that is controlled by China's government.

Dr. Li Meng Yan cited her source as "local doctors." She said: "The description of the market in Wuhan ... is a smokescreen. This virus did not come from nature."

In April, terrified, and carrying only a small amount of luggage, Dr. Yan boarded a flight for Los Angeles. At LA airport she told border authorities her story and pleaded to be allowed to hide as a fugitive in the US.

Meanwhile, her home and office in China were searched, and her loved ones threatened. Her parents were forced to explicitly state explicitly that she is a liar and a traitor. China has since sought to sully her reputation and undermine her claims.

The Wuhan variant contains a loop and four extra amino acids. It is possible that these changes were introduced in the Wuhan lab to study what mutations a bat virus can undergo and to forestall harmful mutations. The highly contagious COVID-19 variant escaped quarantine and was released to the world to perpetrate its harmful actions.

Baker continued:

In 2015 the Wuhan institute performed what is called **"Gain of Function"** experiments– manipulation of viruses in the lab with the intention to exclude infection. These were criticized experiments with the claim that they are dangerous, sensation-gaining but do not show any practical gain.

"I, myself, believe, like Dr. Yan, that what happened was simple. It was an accident. SARS-CoV-2, otherwise known as COVID-19, began its existence inside a bat in a claustrophobic mine shaft, and then it was made more infectious in the Wuhan lab by inserting a piece of RNA. This was a scientist's well-intentioned, but risky effort, to create a broad-spectrum vaccine. SARS COV-2 was not designed as a biological weapon. But it was, designed to produce a harmless variant that will not ever infect humans.

The artificially changed virus spent some time in a laboratory, and one day it was removed from the freezer, was thawed, and the ampule with the mutant fell from the hands of the lab technician or a scientist who was unknown to him became infected. This way the COVID-19 got out.

Other, thoughtful scientists dismiss this notion. They believe that SARS COV-2 arose naturally, "zoonotically," from bats. There was not any study of a bat virus, and it was not hybridized, or sluiced through cell cultures, or otherwise worked on by trained professionals. These scientists hold that a bat, carrying a coronavirus, infected some other creature. They accuse a pangolin, which may have already been sick with a different coronavirus disease. Out of the conjunction and commingling of those two diseases within the pangolin, a new zoonotic virus, highly infectious to humans, evolved. It took only one infected person to cause the pandemic.

There is no direct evidence for this zoonotic turnover possibility. Also, there is no direct evidence for an experimental mishap. No written confession, no incriminating notebook, no official accident report ever was published. Such a mishap certainty craves detail, and investigation. It has been a full year, millions of people have been infected, and, surprisingly, no public investigation has taken place. We still know extraordinarily little about the origins of this disease.

Over the past few decades, scientists have developed ingenious methods of evolutionary acceleration and recombination, and they have learned how to trick viruses, among them also coronaviruses. Scientists have invented machines that mix and mingle the viral codes of bat diseases with the code for human diseases.

Obama White House described this mingling work as "experiments that may be reasonably anticipated to add attributes to Influenza, MERS, or SARS viruses, such that the virus would have (an) enhanced pathogenicity and/or transmissibility in mammals via the respiratory route."

The virologists who carried out these experiments have accomplished amazing feats of genetic transmutation, and there have been very few publicized accidents over the years. But there have been some.

And we were warned, repeatedly. Infectious-disease experts Marc Lipsitch and Thomas Ingles by wrote in 2014 the following: "The intentional creation of new microbes that combine virulence with heightened transmissibility poses extraordinary risks to the public," "A rigorous and transparent risk- assessment process for this work has not yet been established." That is still true today. In 2012. Lynn Klotz in the "Bulletin of the Atomic Scientists" warned that there was an 80 percent chance, given how many laboratories were then handling virulent variants, which a leak of a potential pandemic pathogen would occur sometime in the next 12 years.

A lab accident, a dropped flask, a needle prick, a mouse bite, an illegibly labeled bottle is not something that will be advertised. Proposing that something unfortunate happened during a scientific experiment in a lab is not freely admissible. However, accidents should be reported!

<u>The start of COVID-19's Pandemic</u>

From early 2020, the world was brooding over the origins of COVID-19. People were reading research papers, talking about what kinds of live animals, were or were not sold, at the Wuhan seafood markets — wondering where the new virus had come from.

At the start of the Pandemic, the Chinese government shut down transportation and built hospitals at high speed. There were video clips of people who had suddenly dropped unconscious in the street. A doctor on the U-Tube already told citizens how they were supposed to scrub down produce when we got back from the supermarket.

A scientist wrote in his journal that there seemed to be something oddly artificial about the disease that started in China: "It is too airborne — too catching — it is something that has been selected for infectivity. That is what I suspect. There was no way to know, so therefore there is no reason to waste time thinking about it."

A vast treasure was spent by the U.S. on the amplification and aerial delivery of diseases — some well-known, others obscure and stealthy. America's biological-weapons program in the Fifties had A1-priority status - as high as nuclear weapons. In preparation for total war with a numerically superior communist foe, American scientists bred germs to be resistant to antibiotics and other drug therapies. They infected lab animals with them, using a technique called "serial passaging," to make the germs more virulent and more catching.

And along the way, there were laboratory accidents: By 1960, hundreds of American scientists and technicians had been hospitalized, victims of the diseases they were trying to turn into weapons.

Charles Armstrong, of the National Institutes of Health, one of the consulting founders of the American germ-warfare program, investigated Q fever three times, and all three times, scientists and lab technicians got sick.

In 1951 in the anthrax pilot plant at Camp Detrick, Maryland, a microbiologist, attempting to perfect a "foaming process" of high-volume production, developed a fever and died.

In 1964, veterinary worker Albert Nickel fell ill after being bitten by a lab animal. His wife was not told that he had Matchup virus, (Bolivian hemorrhagic fever). "I watched him die through a little window to his quarantine room at the Detrick infirmary," she said.

In 1977, a worldwide epidemic of influenza A began in Russia and China; it was eventually traced to a sample of an American strain of flu preserved in a laboratory freezer since 1950.

In 1978, a hybrid strain of smallpox killed a medical photographer at a lab in Birmingham, England.

In 2007, live foot-and-mouth disease leaked from a faulty drainpipe at the Institute for Animal Health in Surrey.

In the U.S., "USA Today" printed in an exposé published in 2014 the following: "more than 1,100 laboratory incidents involving bacteria, viruses and toxins that pose significant or bioterror risks to people and agriculture, were reported to federal regulators during 2008 through2012."

In 2015, the Department of Defense discovered that workers at a germ- warfare testing center in Utah had mistakenly sent close to two hundred shipments of live anthrax to laboratories throughout the United States Australia, Germany, Japan, South Korea, and several other countries over the past 12 years.

In 2019, laboratories at Fort Detrick — where "defensive" research involves the creation of potential pathogens were shut down for several months by the Centers for Disease Control and Prevention for "breaches of containment." They reopened in December 2019.

Everyone took sides; everyone thought of the new disease as one more episode in an ongoing partisan struggle. Think of Mike Pompeo, think of Donald Trump himself. They stood at their microphones saying, in a winking, "I- know-something-you-don't-know" sort of way that the COVID-19 disease escaped from a Chinese laboratory. I think that whatever they were saying could be wrong. Anyway, it became impermissible, almost taboo, to admit that covid-19 could have come from a lab accident.

Even high containment laboratories have a whispered history of near misses. Scientists are people, and people have clumsy moments, poke themselves, and get bitten by the enraged animals they are trying to nasally inoculate. Machines can create invisible aerosols, and cell solutions can become contaminated. Waste systems do not always work properly. Things can go wrong in a hundred separate ways.

The story of the COVD-19 disease, as soon as it appeared, was intercepted, and politicized by people with ulterior motives. The basic and extremely interesting scientific question of what happened was sucked up into an ideological quarrel.

Some Americans boycotted Chinese restaurants; others bullied and harassed Asian Americans. Steve Bannon, broadcasting from his living room, in a YouTube series called War Room, said that the Chinese Communist Party had made a biological weapon and intentionally released it. He called it the "CCP virus." And his billionaire friend and backer, Miles Guo, a devoted Trump supporter, told a right-wing website that the communists' goal was to "use the virus to infect selective people in Hong Kong, so that the Chinese Communist Party could use it as an excuse to impose martial law there and crush the Hong Kong pro-democracy movement. But it backfired terribly."

In the Lancet, in February, a powerful counterstatement appeared, signed by twenty-seven scientists. "We stand together to strongly condemn conspiracy theories suggesting that COVID-19 does not have a natural origin," the statement said. "Scientists from multiple countries have published and analyzed genomes of the causative agent, COVID-

19 and they overwhelmingly conclude that this Coronavirus originated in wildlife, as have so many other emerging pathogens."

The behind-the-scenes organizer of this 'Lancet' statement, Peter Daszak, is a zoologist and bat-virus sample collector and the head of a New York nonprofit called Eco Health Alliance — a group that (as veteran science journalist Fred Guterl explained later in 'Newsweek') has channeled money from the National Institutes of Health to Shi Zhengli's laboratory in Wuhan, allowing the lab to carry on recombinant research into diseases of bats and humans. "We have a choice whether to stand up and support colleagues who are being attacked and threatened daily by conspiracy theorists or to just turn a blind eye," Daszak said.

How Did the COVID-19 virus get out? There could be several possibilities:

1. The COVID-19 virus was recovered from Tongguan Mine Shaft by Shi Zhengli's team and transported to the Wuhan Institute of Virology.
2. The Wuhan Institute of Virology, where Shi Zhengli's team brought the RaTG13 bat virus sample, sequenced its genome, then took it out of the freezer several times in recent years.
3. The Wuhan Center for Disease Control and Prevention, which first reported signs of the

COVID-19 coronavirus in hospital patients stored it improperly in its full freezers.

4. The Huanan Seafood Wholesale Market is an early suspected origin of the pandemic, where the first major outbreak occurred.

Vincent Racaniello, a professor at Columbia and a co-host of a podcast called "This Week in Virology," said on February 9 that the idea of an accident in Wuhan was "complete bunk." The coronavirus was 96 percent like a bat virus found in 2013, Racaniello said. "It is not a manufactured virus. It was not released from a lab."

Racaniello's dismissal was seconded by a group of scientists from Ohio State, the University of Pennsylvania, and the University of North Carolina, who put out a paper in "Emerging Microbes and Infections" to quiet the "speculations, rumors, and conspiracy theories that SARS-CoV-2 is of laboratory origin." There was "currently no credible evidence" that SARS-2 leaked from a lab, these scientists said, using a different argument from Racaniello's.

"Some people have alleged that the human SARS-CoV-2 was leaked directly from a laboratory in Wuhan where a bat CoV virus (RaTG13) was recently reported," they said. But RaTG13 could not be the source because it differed from the human SARS-2 virus by more than a thousand nucleotides. One of the paper's authors, Susan Weiss, said: "The conspiracy theory is ridiculous."

The most influential natural-origin article "The Proximal Origin of SARS- CoV-2," published by a group of biologists that included Kristian Andersen of Scripps Research, appeared online in a preliminary version in mid-February. "We do not believe any type of laboratory-based scenario is plausible," the scientists said. Why? Because molecular-modeling software predicted that if you wanted to optimize an existing bat virus so that it would replicate well in human cells, you would arrange things differently than how the COVID-19 virus does it — even though it does an extraordinarily good job of replicating in human cells. "The laboratory-based scenario was implausible," the article said, "because, although it was true that the virus could conceivably have developed its unusual genetic features in a laboratory, a stronger and "more parsimonious" explanation was that the features came about through natural mutation or recombination." "What we think," explained one of the authors, Robert F. Garry of Tulane University, on YouTube, "is that this virus is a recombinant. It came from a bat virus, plus perhaps one of these viruses from the pangolin.

Dr. Fauci dismissed the Wuhan Lab as a Source of Coronavirus. Dr. Fauci said in an interview with National Geographic, the following: "If you look at the evolution of the virus in bats, and what's out there now," Fauci said, "it's very, very strongly leaning toward 'This could not have been artificially or deliberately manipulated. That is the way that mutants naturally evolve."

Recently, a group of French scientists from Aix-Marseille University posted a paper describing their comparison of the base sequence of the Wuhan variant to that of one of the Bat viruses that Shi Zhengli studied (the RaTG13, see above). They confirmed that the two viruses indeed were remarkably similar, with some single base changes. They also said that they detected a peculiar insertion in the genome of the Wuhan strain/variant that is present in the spike protein. This peculiar insertion coded for, are arginine, arginine, alanine, and arginine. It strengthens the "natural origin" of the COVID-19 and negates the "Wuhan human interference" theory.

The genetic composition of the new strain known as the 'Bat Woman' Zhengli, this virologist is considered as one of the world's top researchers on corona virus and has successfully found dozens of deadly SARS-like viruses in bat caves.

Having experience of 16 years in hunting viruses in bat caves, Shi, a researcher at the Wuhan Institute of Virology (WIV), found that the COVID 19 virus originated in bats. According to the "South China Morning Post," the data collected by Shi and her team was brought back to the Wuhan based National Biosafety Laboratory.

According to the website, it was Shi's team which identified that "'the COVID-19 was a direct descendant of a wild strain they culled from the droppings of a fruit bat in Yunnan province. COVID-19 shares 96 per cent of the genes of the bat virus."'

Shi was called back to her lab in Wuhan after the breakout of pandemic at the end of last year. She managed to complete the gene sequencing of COVID-19 within three days. She found that the new strain was associated with horseshoe bats, found in Yunnan. Shi's findings revealed that the COVID-19 was like SARS, a respiratory illness originating from China, which affected thousands of people in 2003.

According to "Scientific American," Shi admitted that when she first called back from a conference to investigate the new unnamed diseases, last year, she feared the possibility of coronavirus escaping her lab. "I wondered if the municipal health authority got it wrong. I had never expected this kind of thing to happen in Wuhan, in central China," she told the science journal.

The Wuhan Institute of Virology (WIV) is located just ten miles from the wildlife sea food market, believed to be the epicenter of coronavirus. Shi said that she finally felt relieved 'after none of the sequences OF COVID-19 matched those of the viruses her team had sampled from bat caves. "That really took a load off my mind. I had not slept a wink for days," she said.

I have supplied you, with enough material to understand that we shall never know what started the plague that we are now under its yoke...

In summary: Whether COVID-19 is a lab-modified virus or not, one thing is certain: Scientists, do not mess with dangerous viruses of bats or of other animals! If you will continue to mess with viruses, we may find ourselves one day with a virus that will completely eradicate humanity!!!!

Chapter 2/1

The recruited post-doctors, their Boss, and the description of the Broad Institute

In a conference room of one of the labs of the **Broad Institute**, sat six young scientists. The conference room was equipped with slide-projector equipment and a long oval conference table with upholstered chairs. In front of the screen of the projecting equipment stood a distinguished-looking gentleman in his late fifties, of medium weight. He wore a suit and sported a black bow tie and a white shirt. His face reflected kindness and compassion and his blue eyes were intelligent. He had a beard and was completely bald. When he met new friends and acquaintances, he liked to joke that he woke up one morning and saw that his scalp hair migrated to his chin. This joke always drew hearty guffaws... This gentleman was a scientist in charge of the lab.

The young scientists did not know each other, as judging by the curious gazes that they directed around.

The Eli and Edythe L. Broad Institute of MIT and Harvard, which housed the conference room and lab where the scientists were, was always referred to as the “Broad Institute.” It is a biomedical and genomic research center located in Cambridge, Massachusetts. The Broad Institute is independently governed and supported as a nonprofit research organization. It is partnered with the Massachusetts Institute of Technology (MIT), Harvard University, and the five Harvard teaching hospitals. The Broad Institute evolved from a decade of research collaborations between MIT and Harvard scientists.

One of the first cornerstones of the Broad Institute was the Center for genome research of the Whitehead Institute at MIT, which was founded in 1982 and became a major center for genomics and the Human Genome Project. As early as 1995, scientists at the Whitehead started pilot projects in genomic medicine. They formed an unofficial collaborative network among young scientists interested in genomic approaches to cancer and human genetics.

Another cornerstone for the 'Broad,' was the Institute of Chemistry and Cell Biology which was established by the Harvard Medical School in 1998to pursue chemical genetics as an academic discipline. Its projecting facility was one of the first high-throughput resources opened in an academic setting. It facilitated small molecule screening projects for more than eighty research groups worldwide.

Next, to create a new organization that was open, collaborative, cross- disciplinary and able to organize projects at any scale, planning took place in 2002–2003. It comprised the institutes described above.

In its first years, philanthropists Eli and Edythe Broad made a founding gift of $100 million when the Broad

Institute was formally launched in 2004. Later, the Broad family announced an additional $100 million gift to the institute and in 2008 they announced an endowment of $400 million to make the Broad Institute a permanent establishment. In 2013, they invested an additional$100 million to fund the second decade of research at the institute. At the start of the Broad Institute, the traditional academic model of individual laboratories working within their specific disciplines could not meet the emerging challenges of biomedicine.

To gain a comprehensive view of the human genome and biological systems, scientists needed to work in a highly integrated fashion. That meant working in nimble teams that combined biology, chemistry, mathematics, computation, and engineering with medical science and clinical research. It also meant working at a scale usually seen more in industry.

Eventually, the Broad Institute needed to foster an atmosphere of creativity, risk-taking, and open sharing of data and research. This new model needed to seek collaborations beyond its borders.

Therefore, it became an "experiment": A new way of doing science in various scientific disciplines. Today, the Broad community contains four thousand scientists, committed to advancing research in areas that include infectious diseases, cancer, psychiatric research, and cardiovascular disease. Each lab has a wide variety of scientists of several disciplines that fertilize each other.

Chapter 2/2

What is the Universal Influenza Vaccine?

The senior scientist in the group that was assembled in one of the libraries of the Broad started its first session, and this is what he said: "Dear colleagues, I am happy to see all of you in my lab in the Broad Institute! In a little while, we shall discuss how we are going to study our project which is the development of a Universal Flu Vaccine.

For easy recognition of all of us, I entered all your names in a chart. I drew this chart for those who remember things better when they see them on paper, or when they are projected, or both. This is a product of their earlier years in school, where they industriously wrote whatever the teachers uttered, sometimes even copying their jokes..."

The elder scientist projected a slide and said:

"This chart will allow you to easily remember information about your colleagues – their names, area of specialization, and their previous Alma Mater:

Name of Post-doctor	Scientific Area	Previous place of post-Doctoring
Harold Kent	Molecular Virology	Department of Microbiology, Harvard medical school
John Appelbaum	Virology	Department of Microbiology, Harvard medical school
Sondra white	Virology and Molecular Genetics	Department of Microbiology, University of Pennsylvania Medical School, Philadelphia, Pa.
Francis Gemmel	Veterinary Virology	School of Veterinary Medicine, Baylor University School of Medicine
Tamara Tabachnick	Molecular Genetics and Protein-Chemistry	John Hopkins school of medicine
Professor John Britten	Virology and Molecular genetics	Department of Microbiology, Harvard medical school

Then the professor said: "Friends! as you know from the enrollment advertisements in the Journal. In my Journals' enrolment-advertisements, I purposely did not mention the subject of our project, in order not to warn any of the potential competitors of our intentions. Some other groups are also working on the development of the Universal Influenza Vaccine.

I shall soon describe to those of you who are not familiar with the subject what it means, although the term is self-explanatory.

There are several groups of scientists who are already working on "our" project. These are:

1) A group in the Rogon research Institute of MIT,
2) NIAID – the National Institute of Allergy and Infectious Diseases,
3) An Immunology team in the University of Chicago,
4) A group in the University of Georgia,
5) A group in the Dana Farber Cancer institute of Harvard Medical School,
6) A group in the Icahn Institute of Medicine of Mount Sinai.

What is the Universal Influenza Vaccine? The vaccine is the "golden fleece" and the "holy grail" of the Influenza (Flu) research. It could free scientists from the often-inaccurate process of predicting the circulating Flu strains of each year and redesigning the vaccine to match them. Unlike some viruses, Influenza shots are required every year due to the large diversity of the Flu viruses, and the variable efficacy of vaccines which are prepared every year to prevent infection. Also, there are antigenic shifts in the Flu which had already created pandemic strains such as the H1N1 outbreak in 2009.

The yearly work to produce the vaccine is a six-month lengthy process. During that time, the virus can mutate, making the vaccines less effective. Also, high risk populations: the elderly and those with chronic diseases, often gain only a limited immunity from the Flu vaccines. The yearly vaccines have been proven to be 30% to 70% effective in preventing hospitalization from the Flu or from pneumonia. On the average, Influenza vaccine's efficacy is 60% among the general population that receive yearly vaccinations.

By creating a Universal Flu vaccine, the need to recreate a yearly shot will be eliminated. The Universal vaccine will provide multi-season and multi- strain protection against all human Influenza virus strains, including also pandemic causing Flu strains. Also, it will be produced in massive quantities and will eliminate the shortage and supply problems of yearly vaccines.

Chapter 2/3

Description of the Influenza virion, its Proteins, and its Nucleic acids

Professor Britten continued: "Let me now project to you on the screen the culprit virus that have claimed so many victims throughout history[23]). Here the professor stopped his talk and a scheme of the virus appeared on the whiteboard:

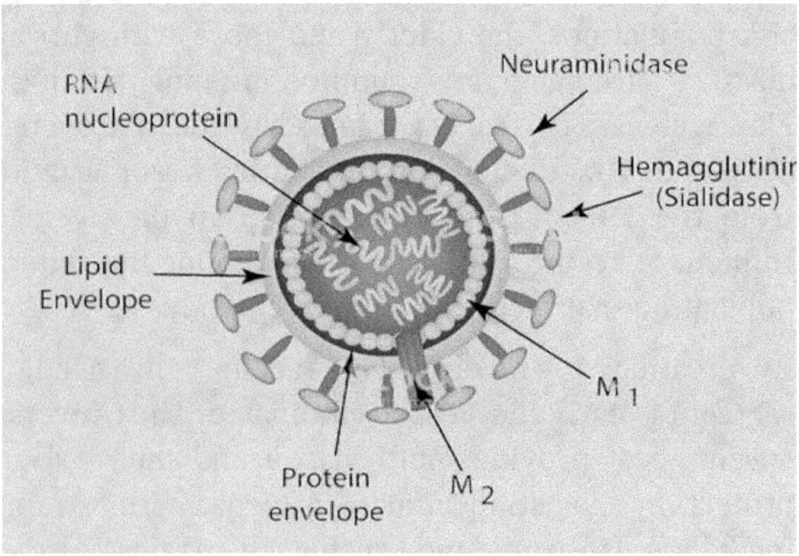

A schematic representation of the Influenza virion (Copyright: Optical Microscopy lab at the National High Magnetic Field laboratory).

---

[23] *I want to interject a personal note: my grandparents on my father's side died in the 1917 pandemic in Poland.*

"When the Flu virus does not cause death, it creates symptoms that may be quite severe, but it does not leave any sequelae. However, the elderly may develop heart problems.

Influenza A, B and C viruses are members of the Orthmyxovirideae, which is a family of enveloped viruses with segmented, single stranded, negative sense RNA as their genome. They are classified by antigenic differences in their nucleoprotein (NP) and matrix protein (M1) which are inside the virion. Influenza A viruses are further classified into 16 hemagglutinin (HA) subtypes (H1–H16) and 9 neuraminidase (NA) subtypes (N1–N9), based on the antigenicity of the HA and NA proteins. All subtypes can be found in their natural reservoir of wild aquatic birds, but they can also infect mammalian species, such as humans, pigs, and horses.

Influenza A viruses cause annual epidemics in humans and occasional pandemics that spread on a global scale with severe consequences for human health. Influenza B viruses naturally infect humans, and occasionally seals, and cause every few years more limited epidemics than Influenza A viruses in humans. Influenza C viruses infect humans and pigs. Sero-epidemiological studies suggested that influenza C viruses a global distribution, although they are clinically benign in humans.

Influenza virions possess a lipid envelope that is acquired during their budding process from the apical plasma- membrane of infected cells. The Flu virion are spherical or ovoid in shape, and their size is 80 to 120 nanometers in diameter. The virions released from infected cells are generally spherical, ranging from 80 to 120 nanometers in diameter. On the other hand, budding virions from the surface of infected cells present as mostly elongated particles, and occasionally also as filamentous particles of uniform diameter. The filamentous forms are more common among some Influenza strains than in others.

The virions are covered with many spikes that are inserted into the viral surface. This feature is common to all viruses (remember the Covid-19, for instance). The HA spikes are rod-shaped, while the NA spikes are mushroom-shaped with a box-shaped head that is connected to the lipid membrane by a stalk. As I have already described before they are the proteins that determine the subtype of Influenza virus (A/H1N1 strain, for example – is Influenza type A with H1- and N1- type spikes).

M1, a peripheral membrane protein that I mentioned a minute ago, is one of the most abundant viral proteins in the virion. It binds to the lipid envelope and is thought to form a layer beneath it to maintain the spherical or filamentous structure of the virion. This lipid envelope is derived from the outer envelope of the infected host-cell, since the newly synthesized virions emerge from it by "budding" and are wrapped with the cell's outer membrane, which they carry on them.

The lipid membrane separates the cell from its environment and compartmentalizes the infected cell's interior molecules. Similarly, they do so also for the virion. The membrane is made of equal weights of protein and lipid, with carbohydrates constituting less than 10 percent.

The lipid membrane of the cell, from which the Influenza virions bud out and carries also serves as regulatory agents in cell growth and adhesion, in addition to their sequestering role.

The Hemagglutinin (HA) spikes are responsible for binding the virion to the infected cell. The name "hemagglutinin" comes from the protein's ability to clump red blood cells (erythrocytes) in vitro ("To agglutinate").

Neuraminidase (NA) spikes, on the other hand, have the properties of an enzyme (as the "ase" at the end of the name suggests). The function of the neuraminidase is: 1) to assist with movement of the Influenza virion through the respiratory tract's mucus, and 2) to assist in the release of the mature virus particles from the infected cells.

In addition to the Hemagglutinin and the Neuraminidase spikes, there are M2 proteins that I described a minute ago which are also embedded in the lipid membrane, and beneath the lipid membrane there are viral proteins called M1, or Matrix proteins. These two M proteins, form a shell around the virion's nucleoprotein. They give additional strength and rigidity to the lipid envelope."

Professor Britten stopped his description of the Flu virion and turned to Harold, one of the young men in the group, and said: "Harold, you are my expert in Molecular Virology. Now is the time for you to describe the viral RNAs (Ribonucleic acids) that are the Nucleic Acids of the virion." Harold Kent, happy to demonstrate his expertise to his fellow scientists, stood up, and said:

"Excuse me if you will find some of my descriptions unclear. You may stop me at any point and ask for clarification.

Influenza A, B, and C viruses are members of the Orthomyxoviridae, which is a family of enveloped viruses with segmented, single-stranded, negative-sense RNA genomes. As already our boss has indicated, The Flu viruses are classified by antigenic differences in their nucleoprotein (NP) and matrix protein (M1), which are present within the virions. Influenza A viruses are further classified into 16 hemagglutinin (HA) subtypes (H1–H16) and 9 neuraminidase (NA) subtypes (N1–N9) based on the antigenicity's of the HA and NA.

Influenza A virions possess a lipid envelope that is acquired from the apical plasma membrane[24])of infected cells during the budding process. The virions

---

[24] *Apical plasma membrane -.the layer of a plasma membrane located toward the inside of the epithelial cells.*

released from infected cells are spherical, ranging from 80 to 120 nm in diameter. On the other hand, budding virions on the surface of infected cells present as mostly elongated particles and occasionally filament to us particles of uniform diameter. As for the spikes of the Flu, the HA spikes are rod-shaped, while the NA spikes are mushroom-shaped with a box-shaped head that is connected to the lipid membrane by a stalk. M1, a peripheral membrane protein, is one of the most abundant viral proteins in the virion. It binds to the lipid envelope and is thought to form a layer beneath it to maintain the spherical or filamentous structure of the virion. The viral genome is enclosed in a shell composed of a layer of M1 protein, HA and NA spikes, and the lipid envelope.

The influenza a virus genome consists of eight segmented, single- stranded, negative-sense RNAs. Each viral RNA (vRNA) segment forms a ribonucleoprotein complex (RNP) together with nucleoproteins and a polymerase complex, which is a fundamental unit for the transcription and replication of the viral genome. Although the exact structure of the intact RNP remains poorly understood, recent electron microscopic studies have revealed certain structural characteristics of the RNP. This review focuses on the findings of these various electron microscopic analyses of RNPs extracted from virions and RNPs inside virions. Based on the morphological and structural observations, I will now summarize the architecture of RNPs within a virion and I will also discuss the genome packaging mechanism by which the vRNA segments are incorporated into virions.

Purified influenza virions visualized by negative staining electron microscopy. The spherical virions, 120 nm in diameter, are covered with spikes composed of HA and NA.

As I already described to you previously, the genomes of influenza A and B viruses consist of eight single-stranded negative-sense RNA segments, while that of influenza C virus consists of seven RNA segments. Each viral RNA (vRNA) segment forms a ribonucleoprotein (RNP) complex which creates a twisted rod-like structure that is folded back and coiled on itself). The whole RNP complexes, and just not the genomic RNA alone, are transcriptionally active. In the RNP complexes, the vRNA is associated with a nucleoprotein (NP) and a heterotrimeric (containing three protein molecules which differ from each other) RNA-dependent RNA polymerase complex.

This heterotrimeric complex is composed of basic polymerase protein 1 (PB1), basic polymerase protein 2(PB2), and acidic polymerase protein (PA). These RNA polymerases are responsible for transcription – synthesis of positive sense segments of vRNA that becomes the RNA of the new virions. The new virions will exocytose from the infected cell which dies.

Within the interior of both the A- and the B- type FLU virions is the viral genome that consists of eight viral

RNA (Ribonucleic Acid) segments. (Flu virus C contains only 7 RNA segments). Each of the 8 RNA segments of the Influenza A or B virus genomes, are about 13,500 nucleotides long.

These RNA segments are linear, negative-sense, single-stranded RNA, with each segment linked to a separate nucleocapsid. These Negative-Sense RNAs are complementary to the positive sense RNA strand which is the protein- coding mRNA-like strand. That means that the negative, single-stranded incoming mRNAs molecules must first be transcribed before they can serve as templates for the translation of the virions' new proteins (with the action of ribosomes). Each RNA segment is in combination with several types of additional proteins that I did not mention before...these are: B1, PB2, PA, NP. The interior of the virion also contains an additional protein called NEP."

Chapter 2/4

The Synthesis of the RNP (Ribonucleoprotein)

Harold now said: "I want to talk now about the RNP (Ribonucleoprotein) and its RNA Dependent RNA Polymerases that I will mention in a minute. These polymerases do two jobs:

1. Transcription (new RNA production) of the negative-sense infecting RNA to a positive-sense complementary RNA that is required for the encoding (translation) of viral proteins.
2. Transcription (replication) of the positive sense RNA into new minus- sense viral RNA molecules for incorporation into new virions for emergence to the outside of the infected cell.

   Although the exact structure of the intact RNP remains poorly understood, recent electron microscopic studies have revealed certain structural characteristics of the RNP: these studies focus on the various electron microscopic analyses of:

   a. RNPs extracted from virions.
   b. RNPs seen inside virions.

Based on these morphological and structural observations, I am going to describe to you the architecture of RNPs within a virion and the genome packaging mechanism by which the vRNA segments are incorporated into virion. As I have previously told you, in the RNP complexes, the vRNA is associated with a nucleoprotein (NP) and a heterotrimeric[25]) RNA-dependent RNA polymerase complex of the basic polymerase protein 1 (PB1), basic polymerase protein 2 (PB2), and acidic polymerase protein (PA).

Unlike most negative-sense RNA viruses, transcription and replication of the influenza virus genome occurs in the nucleus of infected cells. After synthesis of the genomic RNAs and viral proteins, RNPs are also synthesized in the nucleus and exported to the cytoplasm. The transmembrane HA, NA, and M2 proteins are conveyed to the cell surface by the standard exocytic pathway.

The RNPs interact with the M1 proteins and the HA, NA, and M2 proteins at the plasma membrane to be packaged into virus particles. Finally, all the viral components assemble into progeny virions, leading to budding from the apical plasma membrane by membrane fission.

The RNP is the fundamental unit for vRNA synthesis and thus plays key role in the virus life cycle.

Each NP molecule is associated with 20–25 nucleotides of vRNA through its the phosphate-sugar backbone.

---

[25] *Heterotrimeric –a complex of three different proteins bound into a complex. In the case of Influenza –3 different polymerase enzymes*

The NP protein monomer, as observed by negative staining electron microscopy, forms small rods with a length of 6.2 nm and a width of 3.5 nm.

The negatively stained RNPs isolated from virions show twisted rod-like structures and each RNP seems to consist of a single strand of NP monomers. As I already told you, the single-stranded RNA is folded back on itself to give a loop at one end and is coiled on itself to form a double-stranded arrangement except at the loop.

Dear colleagues! The process of the synthesis of RNPs that are the fundamental units for vRNA synthesis and thus play important roles in the virus life cycle is much more complicated. But I will not go into that since it does not contribute to our modification experiments, as I envisage them...

Each NP molecule is associated with 20–25 nucleotides of vRNA through its phosphate-sugar backbone. The vRNA has its nucleotide bases exposed on the outside of the RNP and there are charge interactions between the NP molecules and the phosphate backbone of the vRNA.

NP is the major determinant of the rod-like structure of the RNPs and that the vRNA is wrapped around the NP scaffold.

Harold said: “I think that I will stop here.” He went back to his chair followed by cheers and hand clapping.

Chapter 2/5

The Boss discusses the previous attempts to synthesize a Universal Flu Vaccine

Now the boss retrieved the position near the screen and said: "To develop a Universal Influenza Vaccine is bound to be an exceedingly difficult job because it must protect against many strains and sub-strains of both FLU A and FLU B. These strains and sub-strains contain different hemagglutinins (HA) and have other variabilities, as well.

Now I want to describe to you some of the attempts to produce a Universal FLU Vaccine:

- In 2008, the Acambis Company announced that it is working on a universal Flu vaccine based on the less variable M2 protein component of the Flu virus shell.
- In 2009, the Wistar Institute in the University of Pennsylvania received a patent for using a variety of unspecified peptides" in a Flu vaccine, and announced it was seeking a corporate partner for financing.
- A company by the name of BiondVax identified 9 Conserved epitopes in the PA, PB1, PB2, NP & M1 proteins of the Influenza virus and combined them into a recombinant protein called Multimeric-00. Up to 2020, all seven of Biondvax's completed phase 2 human trials have

> demonstrated safety and significant levels of immunogenicity. Unfortunately, the results of the phase 3 trial failed, and the project was terminated.

Most Flu vaccine consists of inactivated Flu viruses. These viruses are coated with the hemagglutinin (HA), which helps them bind to host cells. After vaccination, the immune system generates squadrons of antibodies that target the HA protein.

These antibodies almost always bind to the head of the HA protein. The head of the HA protein mutates the most rapidly. Parts of the HA stem, on the other hand, very rarely mutate.

One factor that is already known to contribute to antibody preference for the HA head is that the HA proteins are densely clustered on the surface of the virus, so it is difficult for antibodies to access the stem region. The head region is much more accessible.

A new advance has been taken recently: The Center for Disease Control and Allergy (CDC) and other public health laboratories around the world have been sequencing the genes of Influenza viruses since the 1980s. Now the CDC contributed these gene sequences to public databases, such as GenBank external and the Global Initiative Avian Influenza Data (GISAID) to share these sequences by public health researchers. The resulting libraries of gene sequences allow CDC and other laboratories and companies to compare the genes of currently circulating Influenza viruses with the genes of older Influenza virus strains to be used in that year's vaccines. The CDC uses these sequences in order:

- To determine how closely "related" similar Flu virus strains are related to one another genetically.
- To monitor how Flu virus strains are evolving.
- To identify genetic changes that affect the virus' properties.
- For example, to identify the specific changes that are associated with Influenza virus strains that cause them to have high infectivity and to cause more severe disease or to develop resistance to antiviral drugs.
- To assess how well a particular Influenza Flu vaccine might protect against a particular Influenza virus strain based on its genetic similarity to other virus strains.
- To monitor for genetic changes in Influenza viruses circulating in animal populations that could enable them to infect humans (turning zoonotic).

These comparison trees show how closely 'related' individual strains are to one another. Phylogenetic trees of Influenza viruses will usually display how similar a strain's hemagglutinin (HA), or neuraminidase (NA) genes are to one another. Each sequence from a specific Influenza virus has its own branch on the tree. The degree of genetic differences (number of nucleotide differences) between viruses is represented by the length of the horizontal lines (branches) in the phylogenetic tree. The further apart viruses are on the horizontal axis of a phylogenetic tree, the more genetically different the viruses are to one another. It is thought that it is possible that something like the 1918 Flu outbreak could occur again. If a new Influenza strain found its way in the human population, and could be transmitted easily between humans, and caused severe illness.

Hemagglutinin (HA), or neuraminidase (NA) are related to one another. Each sequence from a specific virus type is common also to its Influenza N2). As part of this process, CDC compares the new strain's sequence with the other strain sequences and looks for differences among them. CDC then uses the phylogenetic tree described above to visually represent how genetically different the A(H3N2) strains are from each other. Well, folks, this is what I intended to teach you!"

Chapter 2/6

The epidemiology of the Influenza virus

Professor now turned to John Appelbaum and said: "John! Now is your turn to shine among your colleagues, so that they will realize what an expert you are! From your curriculum vitae I learned that after obtaining your Ph. D., you joined the CDC. I learned that during your stay you participated in the epidemiological study to choose this year's strain for the current vaccine and last years' vaccine!

Please share with us some of your vast epidemiological experience." John stood up and started his narration:

"The CDC is the most advanced players in selecting every year the right strains for a vaccine.

"Dear colleagues, I may repeat some facts that you have already heard from Harold, so I ask your forgiveness for repeating them.

Each year CDC performs whole-genome sequencing on about 7,000 Influenza virus strains from original clinical samples collected through virologic surveillance. We have learned from Harold that an Influenza A or B virus' genome contains eight gene segments that encode the structural virus' twelve proteins, including its important surface proteins: hemagglutinin (HA) and neuraminidase (NA). The Influenza virus' surface proteins determine important properties of the virus, including how the virus responds to certain antiviral drugs, the virus' genetic similarity to current strain(s) of Influenza vaccine viruses, and its potential to confer immunity against zoonotic (animal origin) Influenza viruses.

John said: "Researchers at the NIH's National Institute of Allergy and Infectious Diseases developed an antibody that is capable of recognizing HA stem and was also able to inhibit neuraminidase. Combining that antibody with Tamiflu (an anti-neuraminidase acting drug) helped mice survive a lethal viral challenge.

Genetic variations are important because they affect the structure of an Influenza virus' surface proteins. The substitution of one amino acid for another can affect the properties of a virus, such as how well a virus transmits between people, and how susceptible the virus is to antiviral drugs or current vaccines.

As Harold has already told you, CDC performs genetic characterization of Influenza viruses year-round. This genetic data is used in conjunction with virus antigenic characterization data to help determine which Flu strains should be chosen for the upcoming Northern Hemisphere, or Southern Hemisphere Influenza vaccines. In the months leading up to the WHO vaccine consultation meetings in February and September, CDC collects Influenza viruses through surveillance and compares the HA and NA gene sequences of current vaccine strains against those of circulating Flu viruses.

This is one way to assess how closely related the circulating Influenza strains are to the strains the seasonal Flu vaccine was formulated against. As viruses are collected and genetically characterized, differences can be revealed.

For example, sometimes over the course of a season, circulating viruses will change genetically, which causes them to become different from the corresponding vaccine virus. This is one indication that a different vaccine virus may need to be selected for the next Flu season's vaccine, although other factors, including antigenic characterization findings, heavily affect Flu vaccine decisions. The HA and NA surface proteins of Influenza viruses are recognized by the immune system and can trigger an immune response, including production of antibodies that can block infection.

Antigenic characterization refers to the analysis of a virus's reaction with antibodies to help assess how it relates to another virus.

Over the past five years, CDC has been using "Next Generation Sequencing (NGS)" methodologies, which have expanded the amount of information and detail that sequencing analysis can provide. NGS uses advanced molecular detection (AMD) to identify gene sequences from each virus in a sample. Therefore, NGS reveals the genetic variations among many different Influenza virus particles in a single sample, and these methods also reveal the entire coding region of the genomes. This level of detail can directly benefit public health decision-making in important ways, but data must be carefully interpreted by highly trained experts in the context of other available information.

Chapter 2/7

How is an Influenza Vaccine prepared?

Here professor Britten took the reins of continuous teaching because of the importance of the subject of the Flu vaccine! He started a long treatise on Influenza vaccines. He trusted John, his epidemiologist, but wanted to ensure that the vaccine preparation story is well-covered!

So here is his story which has behind it a lot of glorious scientific work and ensures that a pandemic like that of the pig one in 1917-1918 will never happen again!!!

He said: "New versions of the vaccines are developed twice a year, as the influenza virus rapidly changes. While their effectiveness varies from year to year, most provide modest to high protection against influenza. The United States Centers for Disease Control and Prevention (CDC) estimates that vaccination against influenza reduces sickness, medical visits, hospitalizations, and deaths. Immunized workers who do catch the flu return to work half a day sooner on average. Vaccine effectiveness in those over 65 years old remains uncertain due to a lack of high-quality research. Vaccinating children may protect those around them.

The World Health Organization (WHO) and the US Centers for Disease Control and Prevention (CDC) recommend yearly vaccination for all people over the age of six months, especially those at elevated risk. The European Centre for Disease Prevention and Control (ECDC) also recommends yearly vaccination of high-risk groups. These groups include pregnant women, the elderly, children between six months and five years of age, those with certain health problems, and those who work in healthcare.

The vaccines are safe; fever occurs in five to ten percent of children vaccinated, and temporary muscle pains or feelings of tiredness may occur. In certain years, the vaccine was linked to an increase in Guillain–Barré syndrome[26]) among older people at a rate of about one case per million doses. Although most influenza vaccines are produced using egg proteins, they are still recommended as safe for people who have severe egg allergies. As no increased risk of allergic reaction to the egg-based vaccines has been shown for people with egg allergies. Vaccines produced using other technologies, notably recombinant vaccines and those based on cell culture rather than egg protein), started to become available from 2012 in the US, and later in Europe and Australia. Influenza vaccines are not recommended in those who have had a severe allergy to previous versions of the vaccine itself.

The vaccine comes in inactive and weakened viral forms. The live, weakened vaccine is not

---

[26] *Guillain–Barré syndrome: Guillain-Barré syndrome (GBS) is a rare disorder in which a person's own immune system damages their nerve cells, causing muscle weakness and sometimes paralysis. GBS can cause symptoms that usually last for a few weeks.*

recommended in pregnant women, children less than two years old, adults older than fifty, or people with a weakened immune system. Depending on the type they can be injected into a muscle, sprayed into the nose, or injected into the middle layer of the skin (intradermal. The intradermal vaccine was not available during the 2018–2019 and 2019–2020 influenza seasons.

In the worldwide Spanish flu pandemic of 1918, Pharmacists tried everything they knew, everything they had ever heard of, from the ancient art of bleeding patients, to administering oxygen, to developing new vaccines and serums (chiefly against what we now call Hemophilus influenzae – a name derived from the fact that it was originally considered the etiological agent – and several types of pneumococci) one therapeutic measure, transfusing blood from recovered patients to new victims, showed any hint of success.

In 1931, viral growth in embryonated hens' eggs was reported by Ernest William Good pasture and colleagues at Vanderbilt University. The work was extended to growth of influenza virus by several workers, including Thomas Francis, Jonas Salk, Wilson Smith, and Macfarlane Burnet, leading to the first experimental influenza vaccines. This great victory of its time completely changed the fear from pandemics!

In the 1940s, the US military developed the first approved inactivated vaccines for influenza, which were used in the Second World War. Hen's eggs continued to be used to produce virus used in influenza vaccines, but manufacturers made improvements in the purity of the virus by developing improved processes to remove egg proteins and to reduce systemic reactivity of the vaccine. In 2012, the US Food and Drug Administration (FDA) approved influenza vaccines made by growing virus in cell cultures and influenza vaccines made from recombinant proteins have been approved.

According to the CDC: "Influenza vaccination is the primary method for preventing influenza and its severe complications. Vaccination is associated with reductions in influenza-related respiratory illness and physician visits among all age groups, hospitalization, and death among persons at elevated risk, otitis media among children, and work absenteeism among adults. Although influenza vaccination levels increased during the 1990s, further improvements in vaccine coverage levels are needed.

The egg-based technology (still in use as of 2019) for producing influenza vaccine was created in the 1950s. In the US swine flu scare of 1976, President Gerald Ford was confronted with a potential swine flu pandemic. The vaccination program was rushed yet plagued by delays and public relations problems. Meanwhile, maximum military containment efforts succeeded unexpectedly in confining the new strain to the single army base where it had originated. On that base, several soldiers fell severely ill, but only one died. The program was canceled after about 24% of the population had received vaccinations.

An excess in deaths of twenty-five over normal annual levels as well as four hundred excess hospitalizations, both from Guillain–Barré syndrome, were estimated to have occurred from the vaccination program itself, demonstrating that the vaccine itself is not free of risks. The result can be cited to support lingering doubts about vaccination as well as to counter ungrounded claims about the safety of vaccination. A 2010 study found a significantly enhanced immune response against the 2009 pandemic H1N1 in study participants who had received vaccination against the swine flu in 1976.

A quadrivalent flu vaccine[27]) administered by nasal mist was approved by the FDA in March 2012.

Starting with the 2018-2019 influenza season most of the regular-dose egg- based flu shots and all the recombinant and cell-grown flu vaccines in the United States are quadrivalent. In the 2019–2020 influenza season all regular-dose flu shots and all recombinant influenza vaccine in the United States are quadrivalent.

In February 2020, the FDA approved Fluad Quadrivalent[28]) for use in the United States. In July 2020, the FDA approved both Fluad and Fluad

---

[27]29 *Quadrivalent flu vaccine - A quadrivalent influenza (flu) vaccine is designed to protect against four different flu viruses, including two influenza A viruses and two influenza B viruses.*

[28] *Fluad Quadrivalent – A vaccine for geriatric patients that also contains an adjuvant to increase the antibody response after vaccination with a quadrivalent vaccine.*

Quadrivalent for use in the United States for the 2020–2021 influenza season.

A 2012 meta-analysis found that flu vaccination was effective 67 percent of the time; the populations that benefited the most were HIV-positive adults aged 18 to 55 (76 percent), healthy adults aged 18 to 46 (approximately 70 percent), and healthy children aged six months to 24 months (66 percent).[48] The influenza vaccine also appear to protect against myocardial infarction with a benefit of 15 to 45%.]

Repeated annual influenza vaccination offers consistent year-on-year protection against influenza. There is, however, suggestive evidence that repeated vaccinations may cause a reduction in vaccine effectiveness for certain influenza subtypes; this has no relevance to current recommendations for yearly vaccinations but might influence future vaccination policy. As of 2019, the CDC recommends a yearly vaccine as most studies demonstrate the overall effectiveness of annual influenza vaccination

It takes five to six months for the first supplies of approved vaccine to become available once a new strain of influenza virus with pandemic potential is identified and isolated. These months are needed because the process of producing a new vaccine involves many sequential steps, and each of these steps requires a certain amount of time to complete. The vaccine development process from start (obtaining a virus sample) to end (availability of vaccine for use) is summarized below.

Activities at WHO Collaborating Centers

1. Identification of a new virus: As part of a network set up for surveillance, laboratories around the world routinely collect samples of circulating influenza viruses and submit these to WHO Collaborating Centers for Reference and Research on Influenza for analysis. The first step towards the production of a pandemic vaccine starts when a Centre detects a novel influenza virus that differs significantly from circulating strains and reports this finding to WHO.
   Vaccine virus is grown in eggs because the flu virus grows well in them, and eggs are readily available.

2. Preparation of the vaccine strain (called vaccine virus): The virus must first be adapted for use in manufacturing vaccine. To make the vaccine virus less dangerous and better able to grow in hen's eggs (the production method used by most manufacturers), the virus is mixed with a standard laboratory virus strain and the two are allowed to grow together. After a while, a hybrid is formed which contains the inner components of the laboratory strain, and the outer components of the pandemic strain. It takes three weeks to prepare the hybrid virus.

3. Verification of the vaccine strain: After its preparation, the hybrid virus needs to be tested

to make sure that it truly produces the outer proteins of the pandemic strain, is safe and grows in eggs. Upon completion of this process, which takes another three weeks, the vaccine strain is distributed to vaccine manufacturers.

4. Preparation of reagents to test the vaccine (with reference reagents): In parallel, WHO Collaborating Centers produce standardized substances (called reagents) that are given to all vaccine manufacturers to enable them to measure how much virus they are producing, and to ensure they are all packaging the correct dose of vaccine. This requires at least three months and often represents a bottleneck for manufacturers.

<u>Activities at vaccine manufacturers</u>

1. Optimization of virus growth conditions: The vaccine manufacturer takes the hybrid vaccine virus that it has received from the WHO laboratories, and tests different growth conditions in eggs to find the best conditions. This process requires three weeks.

2. Vaccine bulk manufacture: For most influenza vaccine production, this is performed in nine to twelve-days old, fertilized hen's eggs. The vaccine virus is injected into thousands of eggs, and the eggs are then incubated for two to three

days during which time the virus multiplies. The egg white, which now contains many millions of vaccine viruses, is then harvested, and the virus is separated from the egg white. The partially pure virus is killed with chemicals. The outer proteins of the virus are then purified, and the result is several hundred or thousand liters of purified virus protein that is referred to as antigen, the active ingredient in the vaccine. Producing each batch, or lot, of antigen takes approximately two weeks, and a new batch can be started every few days. The size of the batch depends on how many eggs a manufacturer can obtain, inoculate, and incubate. Another factor is the yield per egg. When one batch has been produced, the process is repeated as often as needed to generate the required amount of vaccine.

3. Quality control: This can only begin once the reagents for testing the vaccine are supplied by WHO laboratories, as described above. Each batch is tested, and the sterility of bulk antigen is verified. This process takes two weeks.

4. Vaccine filling and release: The batch of vaccine is diluted to give the desired concentration of antigen, and put into vials or syringes, and labeled. Then the following parameters are tested:

Sterility, protein concentration and safety by testing in animals. This process takes two weeks.

5. Clinical studies: In certain countries, each new influenza vaccine must be tested in a few people to show that it performs as expected. This requires at least four weeks. In some countries, this may not be required as many clinical trials were done with similar annual vaccine preparation, and the assumption is that the new pandemic vaccine will behave similarly. Clinical testing before approving the vaccine, which adds to the time before the vaccine is available.

The full process, in a best-case scenario, can be completed in five to six months. Then the first final pandemic vaccine lot would be available for distribution and use.

Chapter 2/8

"Sic transit Gloria mundi" ("Thus passes worldly glory"), and the rats, ravens, and cats shall inherit the Earth!"

Professor Britten' steam became deeply knowledgeable on the ins and outs of the Influenza virus because of the excellent summaries that they heard, and they supplemented their knowledge by avid reading of virology textbooks, the professor invited them to a meeting.

At the beginning of the meeting, the Professor looked keen and eager, a had a countenance that was quite different from the one that he usually wore... His post-docs felt that something momentous is about to happen and they were not wrong. Their professor greeted them cursorily and then said:

"Dear friends, today we will start!" His post-docs immediately understood what he meant and started to cheer! Professor Britten smiled and hushed them saying: "Hey, hey, do not jinx the project! It will require many modification experiments by, trial and error, before we succeed, if at all..."

The hushed scientists now wore a serious mien and waited for the boss' words. Professor Britten said:

"My idea will be used for the first experiment that we shall perform. I take this because of my prerogative as your senior colleague... After the performance of my idea, we shall discuss any ideas that you may want to advance.

In my idea, we will produce a "Mega Influenza Vaccine" that will, if we shall succeed, immunize against the most prevalent and virulent strains.

Here is what we shall do: we shall prepare a poly-vaccine that will contain most of the devastating pandemic Flu strains of the past. Both WHO and the CDC have them stored and we shall acquire samples from them and grow them ourselves in human embryonic kidney (HEK) cells.

Each strain will grow separately in its own culture.

Those among you who is not verse in the fine art of tissue culturing envision a series of Petri Plates containing a carpet of cells. But that is not how we going to grow them. Does any of you guys and girls\ know how we are going to do it?"

Tamara Tabachnick raised her hand and said:

"Why, certainly: We shall the cells in spinners or in Bio-reactors, which are big metal walled spinners with air and temperature control." Britten said: You are right! To curtain no. 2 and gather all the goodies there... "

We shall use glass walled spinners that will be placed in 37 degrees centigrade and have an atmosphere of 5% Carbon Dioxide in air and cell growth medium. To those who do not know, a glass-walled type of bio reactor. It has a stirrer that spins the cell growth medium inside the spinner and of cells. The cells are free-floating in medium or are attachment-dependent cell types.

Here is a photograph of a spinner:

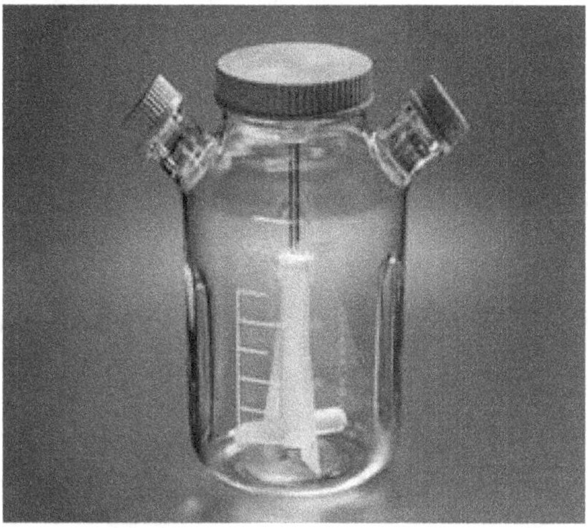

"At the bottom of the spinner there is a vertical magnet. It stirs the culture medium and cells that are in the spinner since the spinner is placed on a magnetic stirrer – a small apparatus that contains another vertical magnet,

The HEK cells that we shall use cannot spin freely in the medium of the spinner. They require attachment to surfaces. The attachment is provided by exceedingly small microcarriers. There are many types of micro carriers, and we will use beads of cross-linked dextran that provide a "natural" substrate for cell growth and allowed improved attachment and spreading of cells with epithelial morphology.

We shall prepare spinners with micro carriers with attached HEK cells. The cells are first grown in a few tissue culture plates and then are removed from the plated with trypsin (a protease enzyme that detaches cells from plates. The cells will be added to packed micro carrier at a bottom of a spinner and allowed to attach. After that medium is added to the spinners and the cells on the micro carrier are spun (mixed) with the magnets,

After the cells grew to a heavy density on the beads, we hall infect the cells in each spinner a different Flu virus. The virus will grow and destroy the cells. The result is a suspension of ready virus.

Next, we shall mix all the virus suspensions in a big vessel to prepare the Mega vaccine with multiple Pandemic Flu strains that we want. Then we shall open the all the flu virions by the addition of Ether which will dissolve the outer coat of the virions. The result will be billions of RiboNucleoProteins (RNPs). These RNPs have a viral RNA bound to, and protected by, the nucleoproteins (NP)!

And voila!!!:We shall have a vaccine remarkably like those RNA vaccines of Pfizer and Moderna!"

The members of the professor's team were stunned at the simplicity of the boss' s idea, and it took several minutes of cogitation before the applauded him.

The team then grew cells in spinners which they bought plus from commercial suppliers that supplied them all the media necessary for the growth of the cells. After of work of 3 weeks' time they had ten liters of a mega-RNA vaccine ready to be tested. Throughout the whole work time they wore heavy protective clothing and masks...

During the preparation of the vaccine the team tried to guess how their boss plans to test their new vaccine. John Appelbaum seemed to the team to suggest the most reasonable proposition – to inject various primates. The team assumed that the Broad institute maintained such primates in their animal houses and John had a glimpse of the houses when he toured through the various buildings of MIT.

During one of the team meetings, John asked Professor Britten:" Hey boss, are we going to use primates for the assay of the safety and efficacy of our vaccine?"

Professor Britten answered: "Oh, I wish we could. But we cannot. We shall have to get permission from the Ethics Committee of the Broad and this is going to take a lot of time because they are swamped with many requests from many Broad labs. We cannot afford to lose any time in this way!!!

Since you already mentioned this point, I shall take this chance to admit the following: I am not so young anymore, I am a widower, and my sons are all grown up. The upshot is that I am going to try the vaccine on myself, and without any additional participants from among you! Here I have a chance to say goodbye to all of you before I will return my soul to the Almighty if it must happen. However, I am confident that it will not happen. History is full of scientists who tried new drugs and vaccines upon themselves. Some of them died but some of them went on to benefit humanity..."

Professor Britten's team tried to dissuade him for a long time, bringing all sorts of arguments. The girl swept and implored their boss, but all to no avail. He kept saying that he wishes to achieve greatness and that no one has the right to take this from him. Finally, the men and women gave-up and sat dejected in the conference room. Harold, who had a paramedics diploma, filled a syringe with the virus and injected Britten into the arm.

Professor Britten finally left for home to lie down, accompanied by Harold. The other men and women of the team set up a watch schedule and brought food for those on vigil and the professor himself. The professor asked whoever watched over him to wear protective equipment and the team complied, but when the professor went to sleep, they took it off.

72 hours of the vigil did not bring any change, but then after the 72 hour the professor woke up with a paroxysm of cough and then lost consciousness, unable to breath

Sondra was on the vigil and immediately requested an ambulance that took him to one of the teaching medical hospitals. At the team's request the professor was put in an isolation ward. It turned out that he had fulminating pneumonia and after 2 hours died without gaining consciousness back!!!All of those who were in contact with the professor followed in his tragic footsteps and from person to person the Flu became more contagious and soon all the rats in the world took control...

Chapter 3/1

The Aspiring residents of the San Francisco's AIDS Foundation

A group of four aspiring interns who just completed their one year of internship, gathered in the library of the HIV & STI[29]) Testing lab of the San Francisco AIDS Foundation. They were going to go through their residency "under the wing" of Dr. Benks. He is an associate professor in the Department of Microbiology of the University of Los-Angeles medical School, and as such was permitted to serve as a mentor for aspiring residents and post-doctoral fellows. Moreover, the Laboratory of the San Francisco AIDS Foundation was affiliated to the medical school as an outpatient clinic and therefore its head could train aspiring residents.

The San Francisco AIDS Foundation is a California nonprofit public benefit corporation which has been granted tax exempt status. It is the biggest AIDS lab in the San-Francisco area.

All four residents, two young men and two young women, completed their internship in St. Luke's Hospital, but because of the COVID-19 plague, they failed to obtain training in the already heavily staffed area hospitals. All San Francisco's hospitals, which treated thousands of corona patients, had all the

---

[29] *STI - -sexually transmitted infections*

personnel that they needed and did not accept any more medical applicants.

Therefore, when they saw an ad asking to fill residents' jobs in HIV & STI Testing lab of the San Francisco AIDS Foundation, which appeared in the 'San-Francisco Chronicle' they immediately applied and were accepted.

They learned that they are going to work and study with Dr. Allan Benks, the head of the San Francisco AIDS Foundation.

As they waited in the reception room, they wondered what kind of a Boss and mentor Dr. Benks is going to be. Is he young or old, strict, or lenient? They were going to undergo 4 year of residency which was going to take place in the Support Department of HIV and AIDS patients during their stint of work and study. Since they were all familiar, with each other, having just completed their internship in St. Luke's Hospital, they discussed their concern together.

Ten minutes later, Dr. Benks entered the room to meet his new aspiring residents. His residents saw a fortyish man with a genuinely nice welcoming smile which dispelled all the apprehensions of his future residents.

Dr. Beck said: "Hi there, my new students and colleagues! I am glad to see you. You were the first to answer my advertisement and therefore you were accepted. It is not that I had many applicants after you. HIV, despite the great advancements in the development of antiviral drugs, still has a dark aura that frightens most people, even advanced medical persons...

During your residency you will work with recovering patients under therapy but fear not! As I am sure, HIV does not spread by the respiratory route like the corona virus! As you may know from the student catalogue of the University of San-Francisco's university, I am an associate professor in the department of Microbiology of the University in addition to my work here in the San Francisco AIDS Foundation. Therefore, I am qualified to be your mentor. I am married and have two children. Now that I have introduced myself, it is your turn to introduce yourselves.

One by one the doctors introduced themselves:

"I am Jack O'reilly, 24 years old and I am veteran surfer."

"I am Florence Jacson, also 24 years old and all my friends call me "Flo" ... I do not like this name because I do not have any flaws, but the name stuck, and I eventually learned to live with it...

"I am Ben Cohen, and I am flutist in the Chamber Orchestra of the San Fracisco University's. I am 26 years old."

"I am Caroline Sala'am, and I serve in my free time as volunteer Paramedic in a local unit of the Red-Cross. I am 25 years old."

Dr. Benks then said: "Well, this will serve for now. I am sure that we will soon learn to recognize each other better. I have also two Residents that are now making the rounds and you can get acquainted later. The chief departmental nurse, Nora, will give you lab-coat, and will assign to you your lockers. I can see that you already carry your stethoscopes in your pockets. Welcome to our humble clinic and I will see you in the afternoon. My chief resident will assign you your duty rosters. So, bye for now." Having carried out his introductory meeting, Dr. Benks hurried to the Antiviral medicines treatment Unit to join the rounds.

Chapter 3/2

Professor Benks describes the properties of HIV, its strains, and the eruption of AIDS

In a first teaching period, Dr. Benks met his students: "Dear students! Before the discovery of anti-HIV excellent medications, the virus was a major frightening scourge.

As you had already learned, HIV (human immune deficiency virus) is a virus that attacks the immune system - the body's natural defense system. Without a strong immune system, the body has trouble fighting off disease. Both the virus and the infection it causes, are called HIV. The HIVs are two species of Lentivirus (a subgroup of retrovirus) that infect humans and are called HIV- 1 and HIV-2. Both these strains can lead to AIDS. However, they are quite different from each other.

Over time, HIV-1 and HIV-2 cause acquired immunodeficiency syndrome (AIDS), a condition in which a progressive failure of the immune system allows life-threatening opportunistic infections and cancers to thrive. Without treatment, the average survival time after infection with HIV is estimated to be 10 to 12 years, depending on the HIV subtype. In most cases, HIV is a sexually transmitted infection and occurs by contact with or transfer of blood, pre-ejaculate fluid, semen, and vaginal fluids.

Research has shown (for both same-sex and opposite-sex couples) that HIV is transmitted through condom-less sexual intercourse, even if the HIV- positive partner has a consistently undetectable viral load.

Non-sexual transmission can occur from an infected mother to her infant during pregnancy, during childbirth by exposure to her blood or vaginal fluid, and through breast milk. Within these bodily fluids, HIV is present as both free virus particles and as a virus within infected immune cells.

White blood cells are an important part of the immune system. HIV infects and destroys white blood cells called CD4+ cells. If too many CD4+ cells are destroyed, the body can no longer defend itself against infection.

The last stage of HIV infection is AIDS. People with AIDS have a small number of CD4+ cells and get infections or cancers that rarely occur in healthy people. These can be deadly. But having HIV does not mean you have AIDS. As I already told you, even without treatment, it takes a long time for HIV to progress to AIDS—usually 10 to 12 years.

When HIV is diagnosed before it becomes AIDS, medicines can slow, or stop even more, the damage to the immune system. If AIDS does develop, medicines can often help the immune system return to a healthier state. With treatment, many people with HIV can live long and active lives.

As I already described, there are two main types of human immune deficiency virus (HIV): HIV-1 and HIV-2. Both can lead to AIDS. However, they are quite different from each other.

HIV-1 is the most common type. When you hear the term "HIV," it is HIV-1.

HIV-2 occurs in a much smaller number of people, mostly in West Africa. In the U.S., it makes up only 0.01% of all HIV cases, and those are primarily people from West Africa. It is harder to transmit HIV-2 from person to person, and it takes longer for the infection to turn into AIDS. Both HIV-1 and HIV-2 have multiple groups within them. Those groups branch out even further into subtypes, or strains.

HIV constantly makes copies of itself. Some strains multiply faster and can be passed from person to person more easily than others. A doctor can treat HIV better if he knows what strain you have. The type of HIV can be tested by a blood test that also can tell if certain HIV drugs will not work well for you.

HIV-1 has four **groups** -- one large one and three much smaller ones. These are: M, N, O, and P.

Group M (Major) - This group was responsible for HIV epidemics. 90% of all HIV-1 cases stem from this group. The group has nine named strains: **A, B, C, D, F, G, H, J, and K.** some of these have sub-strains. Researchers find new strains all the time as they learn more about HIV-1 **group** M.

The **group** M's / B strain is the most common in the U.S. Worldwide, the most common HIV **strain** is **C.**

Scientists have not done much research on **strains** other than **B,** so information on the rest is limited. The drugs that treat the **B strain** (antiretroviral drugs) also work on most others.

The smaller HIV-1 groups are rare outside of west central Africa, specifically Cameroon. They are:

Group N: This form of the virus has only been seen in a small group of people in Cameroon. Researchers have not named any strains for this group because there are so few cases of it.

Group O: This group has as many variations as the M group. However, researchers have not identified its separate strains yet, because it is so rare.

Group P: This is the newest group of HIV-1. It was given its own name because of how different it is from the M, N, and O strains.

Infections with Multiple Strains

When the virus multiplies, the copies sometimes change (mutate) and develop into another HIV strain in a patient's body. The patient can end up with a strain that HIV drugs will not work against. This makes the patient's viral load - the amount of HIV in the body - go up. In that case, another type of treatment is needed.

A patient can also have two or more strains if more than one person infected him. This is called super infection. Super infection is rare -- it happens in less than 4% of people. A patient is at the highest risk of super infection in the first 3 years after contracting HIV.

What are the symptoms of HIV and AIDS?

"HIV may not cause symptoms early on. People who do have symptoms may mistake them for the Flu or mononucleosis. Common early symptoms include Fever, sore throat, Headache, Muscle aches and joint pain, swollen glands (swollen lymph nodes), Skin rash.

Symptoms may appear from a few days to several weeks after a person is first infected. These early symptoms usually go away within 2 to 3 weeks.

After the early symptoms go away, an infected person may not have symptoms again for many years. After a certain point, symptoms reappear and then remain. These symptoms usually include swollen lymph nodes, Extreme tiredness, Weight loss, Fever, Night sweats.

How can one prevent HIV?

Dear Colleagues!

San Francisco has a higher frequency of HIV than most cities in our country. As such, I want you, whenever you can act as counselors and tell your acquaintances and your patients in the clinic the following measures against HIV infections: HIV is often spread by people who do not know they have it. So, it is always important to protect yourself and others by taking these steps:

Practice safer sex. Use a condom every time you have sex (including oral sex) until you are sure that you and your

Tell your acquaintance that a doctor may suspect HIV if symptoms last and no other cause can be found. If a person has been exposed to HIV, his body will make antibodies to destroy the virus. Doctors use tests to find these HIV antibodies or antigens in urine, saliva, or blood. If a test on urine or saliva shows that a person is infected with HIV, he will have a blood test to confirm the results. Most doctors strait-away use a blood test to diagnose HIV infection. If the test is positive (meaning that HIV antibodies or antigens are found), a test to detect HIV DNA or RNA will be done to be sure. HIV antibodies or antigens usually show up in the blood within 3 months. If a person, man, or a woman think that they have been exposed to HIV, but their first test is negative, they should be tested again. A repeat test may be done after a few weeks to be sure you are not infected.

HIV infects vital cells in the human immune system, such as helper T cells (specifically CD4+Tcells), macrophages, and dendritic cells. HIV infection leads to low levels of CD4+ T cells through several mechanisms, including pyroptosis[30]) of abortively infected T cells, apoptosis[31]) of uninfected bystander cells, the direct viral killing of infected cells, and killing of infected CD4+ T cells by CD8+ cytotoxic lymphocytes that recognize infected cells. When CD4+ T cell numbers decline below a critical level, cell-mediated immunity is lost, and the body becomes progressively more susceptible to opportunistic infections, leading to the development of AIDS".

---

[30] *Pyroptosis - It is also a form of regulated necrosis, is a lytic type of cell death inherently associated with inflammation. It is mediated by the catalytic activity of enzymes called "inflammatory caspases."*

[31] *Apoptosis – Also called programmed cell death. The death of cells which occurs as a normal and controlled part of an organism's growth or development or pathologic process.*

Chapter 3/3

The life cycle of HIV and how its Nucleic Acids and Proteins are synthesized

Dr Benks continued 'to instruct his students and showed them a scheme depicting the life cycle of the HIV:

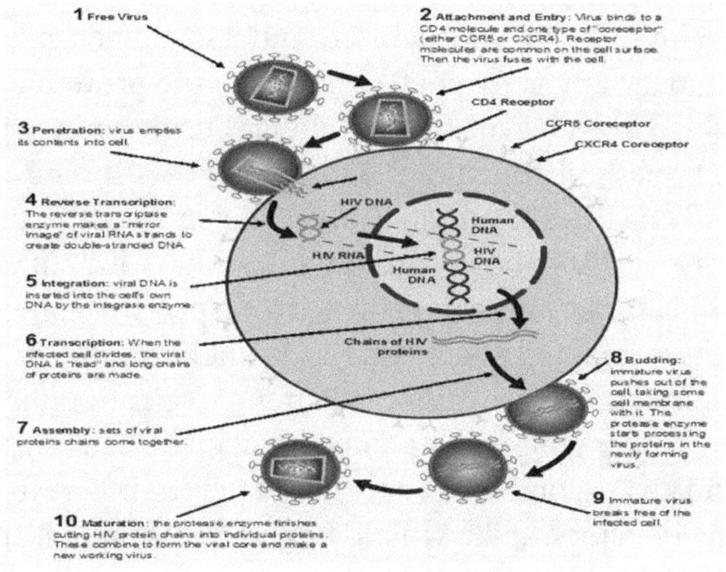

COPYRIGHT: AIDS info net

Then he said "A significant role in the attachment of HIV to CD4 T cells is played by Envelope glycoprotein gp120 which is a glycoprotein exposed on the surface of the HIV envelope. The 120 in its name comes from its molecular weight of 120 kiloDalton. Gp120 is essential for virus entry into cells as it plays a vital role in attachment to specific cell surface receptors.

These receptors are DC-SIGN Heparan Sulfate Proteoglycan and the CD4 receptor on helper T-cells. Binding to CD4 induces the start of a cascade of conformational changes in gp120 and gp41 that lead to the fusion of the viral membrane with the host cell membrane. Binding to CD4 is electrostatic, although there are van der Waals interactions and hydrogen bonds.

Gp120 is coded by the HIV env gene, which is around 2.5 kb long and codes for around 850 amino acids. The primary env (envelope) product is the protein gp160, which gets cleaved by the cellular Furin protease in the endoplasmic reticulum[32]) to gp120 (~480 amino acids) and gp41 (~345 amino acids). The crystal structure of core gp120 shows an organization with an outer domain, an inner domain with respect to its termini and a bridging sheet. Gp120 is anchored to the viral membrane, or envelope, via non-covalent bonds with the transmembrane glycoprotein, gp41. Three gp120s and gp41s combine in a trimer of heterodimers to form the envelope spike which mediates attachment to and entry into the host cell. Most viral structural proteins are components for the capsid and the envelope of the virus. The genetic material of a virus is stored within a viral protein structure called the capsid. The capsid is

[32] *Endoplasmic reticulum -It is a network of membranous tubules within the cytoplasm of a eukaryotic cell, continuous with the nuclear membrane. It usually has ribosomes attached and is involved in protein and lipid synthesis.*

a “shield” that protects the viral nucleic acids from getting degraded by host enzymes.

Dear colleagues, below I picked from the Wikipedia a scheme showing the RNA of the virus as it enters the cell. It describes the location of the various genes – the GAG, POL, ENV, TAT, VPU and REV plus the structural, envelope and accessory proteins that they code.

It is a complicated scheme that you are not asked to memorize, and it will not appear as a question in your final residency exam...

<u>Structure of the genome of the HIV:</u>

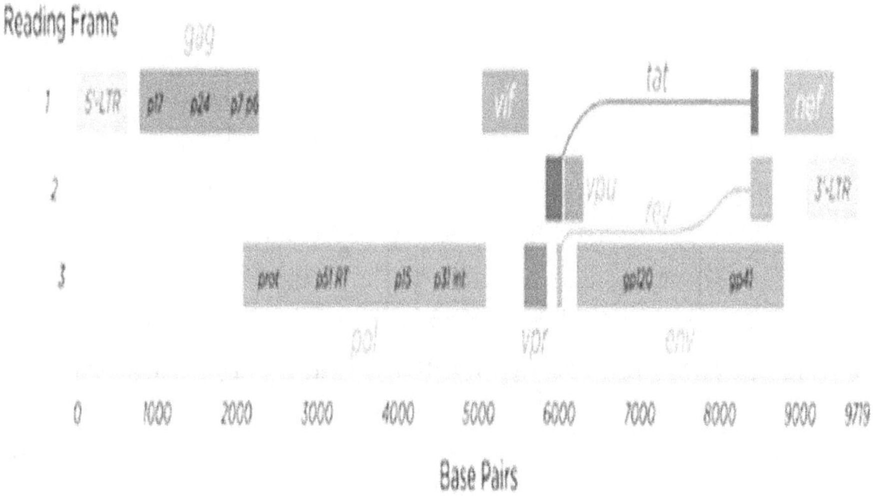

The seven stages of the HIV life cycle are: 1) <u>binding</u>, 2) <u>fusion</u>, 3) <u>reverse transcription</u>, 4) <u>integration</u>, 5) <u>replication</u>, 6) <u>assembly</u>, and 7) <u>budding</u>. To understand each stage in the HIV life cycle, it helps to first imagine what HIV looks like.

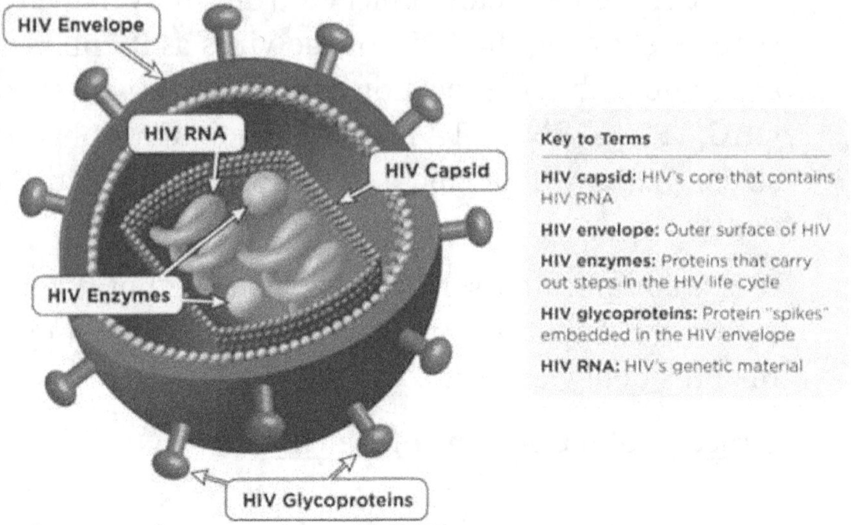

What are the proteins of HIV?

The proteins of HIV are synthesized as polyproteins which produce proteins for virion interior, called Gag, group specific antigen; the viral enzymes (Pol, polymerase) or the glycoproteins of the virion env (envelope). In addition to these, HIV encodes for proteins which have certain regulatory and auxiliary functions as well. These are synthesized as polyproteins which produce proteins for virion interior, called Gag, group specific antigen; the viral enzymes (Pol, polymerase) or the glycoproteins of the virion env (envelope). In addition to these, HIV encodes for proteins which have certain regulatory and auxiliary functions as well.

Dr. Benks continued: "Dear colleagues! I want now to describe the stages of the HIV life cycle in greater detail."

1. Binding

This is the very first stage of the HIV Life cycle. The HIV virus attacks the CD4 cell[33]) and attaches itself to the cell on its surface. It does this by first attaching to the CD4 cell's receptor and then to the CCR5 or the CXCR4 co receptor.

2. Fusion

The second stage of the HIV life cycle is called fusion, and this is done after the virus has effectively attached itself to the CD4 cell. The entire HIV viral envelope will then fuse with the cell which allows it to enter it.

3. Reverse Transcriptase

The third stage happens once the HIV virus has entered the CD4 cell. This allows the virus to release an HIV Enzyme - or reverse transcriptase, enabling it to convert the virus's genetic makeup. It converts the HIV RNA to HIV DNA. This conversion is what allows the HIV Virus to enter the cell's nucleus to integrate with it.

---

[33] *CD4 receptor: A protein present on the outside of infection-fighting white blood cells. CD4 receptors allow HIV to bind to and enter cells. Co-receptor: In addition to binding to a CD4 receptor, HIV must also bind either a CCR5 or CXCR4 co-receptor. CD4 cells are types of white blood cell that detect and fights foreign invaders of the body.* They carry *the CD4 receptor on their surface.*

4. Integration

When the HIV virus has successfully entered the CD4 cell's nucleus it releases another HIV enzyme known as integrase. This is the enzyme the virus uses to integrate its own DNA into the infected CD4 cells DNA. This is the fourth step in the HIV virus life cycle.

5. Replication

The fifth stage of the HIV life cycle is when the virus starts to form long chains of HIV proteins. `These are the protein chains that the HIV virus uses to replicate itself and spread to other CD4 cells in the body.

6. Assembly

The sixth stage of the HIV virus life cycle is when the new HIV RNA and proteins which are now produced by the infected CD4 cell make their way to the surface of the cell to assemble into noninfectious immature HIV.

7. Budding

The final stage of the HIV life cycle is when the immature HIV is released from within the infected CD 4 that produced it. Being an immature HIV, it is unable to infect another CD4 cell, so it releases another HIV enzyme known as a protease. The function of this enzyme is to break up the long chains of proteins forming the immature HIV. Once separated they then combine and mature into the infectious form of HIV.

Now follow in the scheme that I have just screened. Each stage in the HIV life cycle is shown from the start in HIV attacks a CD4 cell and then uses the cell machinery to multiply:

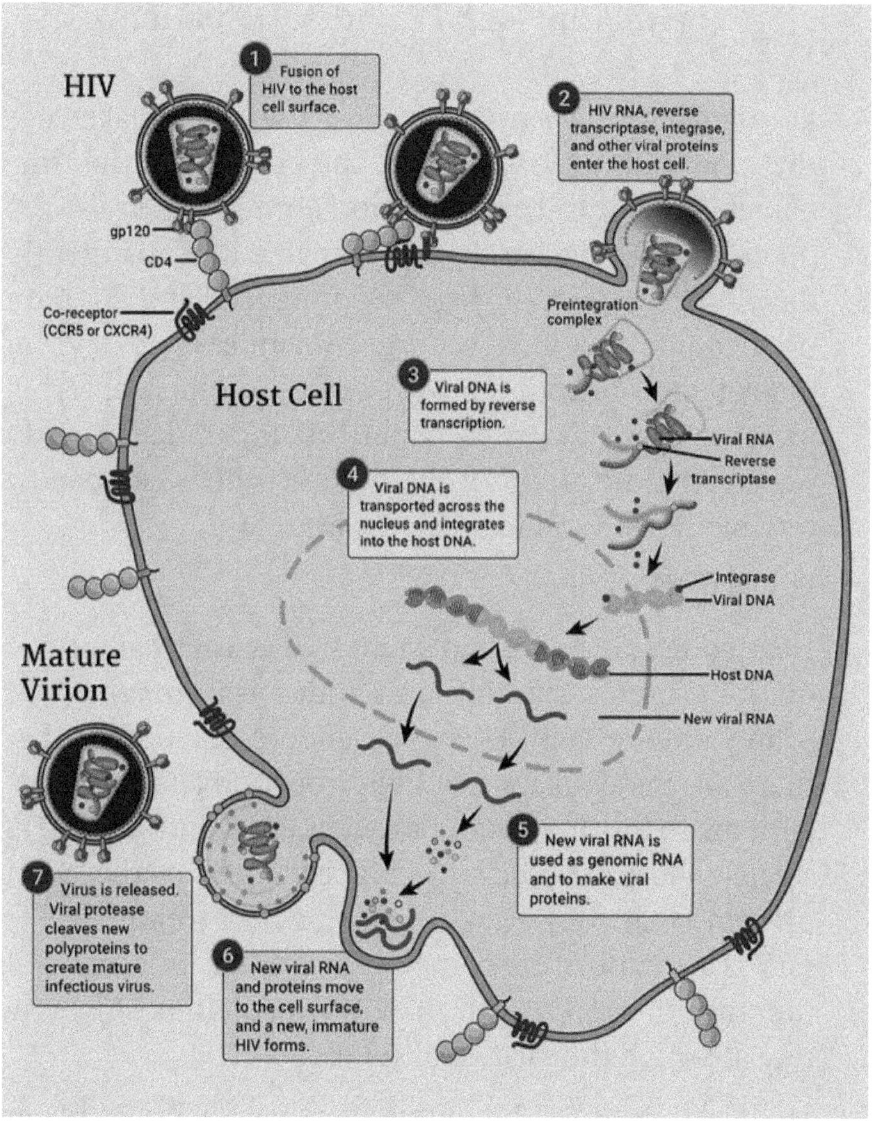

Chapter 3/4

The therapy of HIV and AIDS patients

Dr. Benks said: Dear Colleagues! I want to make sure that you will not be afraid of the HIV when the time comes for you to treat patients. I am going to list the phenomenally successful drugs that had been urgently developed to ensure that HIV infection and AID, do not become a national scourge! So, unless you have an unprotected encounter with any of the just entering patients, Ha, Ha! which is not recommended, you do not have to be afraid of the disease which had been a terrible stigma and fear in the past...

How is HIV treated?

Dear colleagues! It is important to learn all that we can on the proteins that the virus codes as it infects a cell – an immune cell! Then you should remember that there are many drugs that fight infection and help HIV patients to live longer and prevent entry into the AIDS stage. These are classified according to the viral proteins that they attack. The standard treatment for HIV is a combination of medicines called antiretroviral therapy, or ART. Antiretroviral medicines slow the rate at which the virus multiplies.

Medical experts recommend that people begin treatment for HIV as soon as they know that they are infected.

To monitor the HIV infection and its effect on a person's immune system, a doctor will regularly do two tests:

Viral load, which shows the amount of virus in your blood and a CD4+ cell count, which shows how well your immune system is working.

After a patient starts treatment, it is important for him to his medicines exactly as directed by his doctor. When treatment does not work, it is often because HIV has become resistant to the medicine. This can happen if a patient does not take his medicines correctly.

What are the antiretroviral medicines? (Copied from the Wikipedia)

Dear readers! This section on the antiretroviral medicines should apply only to very few of my readers (if I will have any readers at all...At any rate if there will be readers who may be tempted to perform unprotected sex on the assumption that HIV infection can be readily treated, PLEASE DO NOT BE LURED!!!! If you are promiscuous, you may infect innocent partners even if your viral load is undetectable!!!

The management of HIV/AIDS normally includes the use of multiple antiretroviral drugs to control infection. There are several classes of antiretroviral agents that act on various stages of the HIV life cycle. The use of multiple drugs that act on different viral targets is known as highly active antiretroviral therapy (HAART). HAART decreases the patient's total burden of HIV, maintains function of the immune system, and prevents opportunistic infections that often lead to death. HAART also prevents the transmission of HIV between Sero discordant[34]) same sex and opposite sex partners, so long as the HIV-positive partner maintains an undetectable viral load.

Treatment has been so successful that in many parts of the world, HIV has become a chronic condition in which progression to AIDS is increasingly rare. Anthony Fauci, head of the United States National Institute of Allergy and Infectious Diseases, has written, "With collective and resolute action now and a steadfast commitment for years to come, an AIDS-free generation is indeed, within reach." In the same paper, he noted that an estimated 700,000 lives were saved in 2010 alone by antiretroviral therapy.

The United States Department of Health and Human Services and the World Health Organization recommend offering antiretroviral treatment to all patients with HIV. Because of the complexity of selecting and following a regimen, the potential for side effects, and the importance of taking medications regularly to prevent viral resistance, such organizations emphasize the importance of involving patients in therapy choices and recommend analyzing the risks and the potential benefits.

---

[34] *Sero discordant – also known as "mixed status," where one partner is infected by HIV and the other partner is not.*

The World Health Organization has defined health as more than the absence of disease. For this reason, many researchers have dedicated their work to better understanding the effects of HIV-related stigma, the barriers it creates for treatment interventions, and the ways in which those barriers can be circumvented.

Description of the mechanism of the four classes of available antiretroviral drugs against HIV

There are four classes of drugs, which are usually used in combination, to treat HIV infection. Antiretroviral (ARV) drugs are broadly classified by the phase of the retrovirus life cycle that the drug inhibits. Typical combinations include two nucleoside reverse-transcriptase inhibitors (NRTI) as a "backbone" along with one non-nucleoside reverse-transcriptase inhibitor (NNRTI), protease inhibitor (PI) or integrase inhibitors (also known as integrase nuclear strand transfer inhibitors or INSTIs) as a "base."

Nucleoside/nucleotide reverse-transcriptase inhibitors

Nucleoside reverse-transcriptase inhibitors (NRTI) and nucleotide reverse- transcriptase inhibitors (NtRTIs) are nucleoside and nucleotide analogues which inhibit reverse transcription. HIV is an RNA virus, so it cannot be integrated into the DNA in the nucleus of the human cell unless it is first "reverse" transcribed into DNA. Since the conversion of RNA to DNA is not naturally done in the mammalian cell, it is performed by a viral protein- reverse transcriptase, which makes it a selective target for inhibition. NRTIs are chain terminators. Once NRTIs are incorporated into the DNA chain, their lack a 3' OH group prevents the subsequent incorporation of other nucleosides. Both NRTIs and NtRTIs act as competitive substrate inhibitors.

Examples of NRTIs:

Zidovudine, Abacavir, Lumivudine, Emtricitabine, and of Nt tenofovir and Aadefovir.

Non-nucleoside reverse-transcriptase inhibitors

Non-nucleoside reverse-transcriptase inhibitors (NNRTI) inhibit reverse transcriptase by binding to an allosteric site of the enzyme; NNRTIs act as non-competitive inhibitors of reverse transcriptase. NNRTIs affect the handling of substrate (nucleotides) by reverse transcriptase by binding near the active site. NNRTIs can be further classified into 1st generation and 2nd generation NNRTIs. 1st generation NNRTIs include Nevirapine and Efavirenz. 2nd generation NNRTIs are Rrilpivirine. HIV-2 is naturally resistant to NNRTIs.

Integrase inhibitors

Integrase inhibitors (also known as integrase nuclear strand transfer inhibitors or INSTIs) inhibit the viral enzyme integrase, which is responsible for integration of viral DNA into the DNA of the infected cell. There are several integrase inhibitors under clinical trial, and

Raltegravir became the first to receive FDA approval in October 2007. Raltegravir has two metal binding groups that compete for substrate with two Mg2+ ions at the metal binding site of integrase. As of early 2014, two other clinically approved integrase inhibitors are Elvitegravir and Dolutegravir.

Protease inhibitors

Protease inhibitors block the viral protease enzyme necessary to produce mature virions upon budding from the host membrane. Particularly, these drugs prevent the cleavage of gag and gag/pol precursor proteins. Virus particles produced in the presence of protease inhibitors are defective and mostly non-infectious. Examples of HIV protease inhibitors: Lopinavir, Indinavir, Nelfinavir, Amprenavir and Ritonavir. Darunavir and Atazanavir are recommended as first line therapy choices. Maturation inhibitors have a similar effect by binding to gag, but development of two experimental drugs in this class, Bevirimat and Vivecon, was halted in 2010. Resistance to some protease inhibitors is high. Second generation drugs have been developed that are effective against otherwise resistant HIV variants.

Combination therapy

The life cycle of HIV can be as short as about 1.5 days from viral entry into a cell, through replication, assembly, and release of additional viruses to infection of other cells. HIV lacks proofreading enzymes to correct errors made when it converts its RNA into DNA via reverse transcription.

Its short life cycle and high error rate cause the virus to mutate very rapidly, resulting in a high genetic variability. Most of the mutations either are inferior to the parent virus (often lacking the ability to reproduce at all) or convey no advantage, but some of them have a natural selection superiority to their parent and can enable them to slip past defenses such as the human immune system and antiretroviral drugs.

The more active copies of the virus, the greater the possibility that one resistant to antiretroviral drugs will be made.

When antiretroviral drugs are used improperly, multi-drug resistant strains can become the dominant genotypes very rapidly. In the era before multiple drug classes were available (pre-1997), the reverse-transcriptase inhibitors Zidovudine, Didanosine, Zalcitabine, Stavudine, and Lamivudine were used serially or in combination leading to the development of multi-drug resistant mutations.

In contrast, antiretroviral combination therapy defends against resistance by creating multiple obstacles to HIV replication. This keeps the number of viral copies low and reduces the possibility of a superior mutation.

If a mutation that conveys resistance to one of the drugs arises, the other drugs continue to suppress reproduction of that mutation. With rare exceptions, no individual antiretroviral drug has been demonstrated to suppress an HIV infection for long; these agents must be taken in combinations to have a lasting effect.

As a result, the standard of care is to use combinations of anti- retroviral drugs. Combinations usually consist of three drugs from at least two different classes. This three-drug combination is commonly known as a triple cocktail. Combinations of anti retrovirals are subject to positive and negative synergies,[35]) which limits the number of useful combinations.

Because of HIV's tendency to mutate, when patients who have started an antiretroviral regimen fail to take it regularly, resistance can develop. On the other hand, patients who take their medications regularly can stay on one regimen without developing resistance. This greatly increases life expectancy and leaves more drugs available to the individual should the need arise.

---

[35] *Positive and negative synergies - Synergistic effects may be negative or positive, we can say it either synergy or dysergy based on its effect. "An idea that the whole is greater or lesser than that the sum of its parts." It helps to develop competencies. Synergy is also known as "Positive Synergy." Origin of word synergy: Derived from Greek word "synergos".*

In recent year, drug companies have worked together to combine these complex regimens into single-pill fixed-dose combinations. More than twenty antiretroviral fixed-dose combinations have been developed.

This increases the ease with which they can be taken, which in turn increases the consistency with which medication is taken, and thus their effectiveness over the long-term. One day, Dr. Benks, in a meeting, asked his pupils: "Dear colleagues, who can tell me that he read on experiments designed to produce a HIV vaccine or vaccines?

The aspiring interns thought hard, and no one knew the answer. Suddenly Flo raised her hand and when she received permission to talk, said:

"Hey, there is no need to prepare a vaccine given the fact that there are so many Anti-retroviral medicines, so that it is unnecessary to create a vaccine. Besides, it will have to be a polyvalent vaccine for the various current strains..."

The professor as happy with Flo's answer and told her to go to curtain no. 3 and gather all the goodies there...

Chapter 3/5

The attempts to modify the HIV

One day, Dr. Benks, in a meeting, asked his pupils: "Dear colleagues, who can tell me that he read on experiments designed to produce a HIV vaccine or vaccines?

The aspiring interns thought hard, and no one knew the answer. Suddenly Flo raised her hand and when she received permission to talk, said:

"Hey, there is no need to prepare a vaccine given the fact that there are so many Anti-retroviral medicines, so that it is unnecessary to create a vaccine. Besides, it will have to be a polyvalent vaccine for the various current strains..."

The professor as happy with Flo's answer and told her to go to curtain no. 3 and gather all the goodies there...

Chapter 4A/1

The Ebola virus

The genera Ebola virus and Marburg virus were originally classified as the species of the now-obsolete genus Filo virus. In March 1998, the Vertebrate Virus Subcommittee proposed in the International Committee on Taxonomy of Viruses (ICTV) to change the genus Filo virus to the family Filoviridae with two specific genera: Ebola-like viruses and Marburg-like viruses. This proposal was implemented in Washington, D.C., as of April 2001 and in Paris as of July 2002. In 2000, another proposal was made in Washington, D.C., to change the "-like viruses" to "-virus" resulting in today's Ebola virus and Marburg virus.

The first known Ebola outbreaks in humans struck simultaneously in the Republic of the Sudan and the Democratic Republic of Congo in 1976. Ebola is spread through contact with blood or other body Fluids, or tissue from infected people or animals. The known strains vary dramatically in their deadliness,

The mortality rate in the first outbreak was 25%, but, according to the World Health Organization (WHO), it was 90% in the 1998-2000 outbreak in the Democratic Republic of Congo, as well as in the 2005 outbreak in Angola, the five characterized species of the genus Ebola virus are as follows:

A. Zaire Ebola virus (ZEBOV)

Also known simply as the Zaire virus, ZEBOV has the highest case-fatality rate, up to 90% in some epidemics, with an average case fatality rate of approximately 83% over 27 years. There have been more outbreaks of Zaire Ebola virus than of any other species. The first outbreak took place on 26 August 1976 in Yambuku, (the northern Democratic Republic of the Congo), about one hundred kilometers from the Ebola River. This is how the Zaire virus was named. It gave also eventually the name to the five species of the Genus Ebola virus. The symptoms of the virus resembled malaria, and subsequent patients received quinine. Transmission has been attributed to reuse of unsterilized needles and close personal contact. The virus is responsible for the 2014 West Africa Ebola virus outbreak, with the largest number of deaths to date.

B. Sudan Ebola virus (SUDV)

Like ZEBOV, SUDV emerged in 1976; it was at first assumed to be identical with ZEBOV. SUDV is believed to have broken out first amongst cotton factory workers in Nzara, South Sudan, in June 1976. Scientists tested local animals and insects in response to this; however, none tested positive for the virus. The carrier is still unknown. The lack of "bedside isolation" facilitated the spread of the disease. The average fatality rates for SUDV were 54% in 1976, 68% in 1979, and 53% in 2000 and 2001.

C. Reston Ebolavirus (RESTV)

This virus was discovered during an outbreak of simian hemorrhagic fever virus (SHFV) in macaque monkeys from Hazleton Laboratories, in Covance. The laboratory belongs to a contract research organization (CRO) with headquarters in Princeton, New Jersey. Since the initial outbreak in Reston, Virginia, it has since been found in nonhuman primates in Pennsylvania, Texas, and Siena, Italy. In each case, the affected animals had been imported from a facility in the Philippines, where the virus has also infected pigs. Despite its status as a Level 4 virus and its apparent pathogenicity in monkeys, RESTV did not cause disease in exposed human laboratory workers.

D. Tai Forest Ebolavirus (TAFV)

Formerly known as "Ivory coast Ebolavirus," it was first discovered in 1994 among chimpanzees from the Tai Forest in Côte d'Ivoire, (Ivory Coast) Africa. Autopsies had shown that blood within the heart to be brown and no obvious marks were seen on the organs. Also, one autopsy displayed lungs filled with blood. Studies of tissues taken from the chimpanzees showed results seen in human cases from the 1976 Ebola outbreaks in Zaire and Sudan. As more dead chimpanzees were discovered, many of them tested positive for Ebola using molecular techniques. The source of the virus was believed to be the meat of infected western red Colo bus monkeys. One of the scientists performing the autopsies on the infected chimpanzees, contracted Ebola. She developed symptoms like those of dengue fever a week after the autopsy and was transported to Switzerland for treatment. She was discharged from the hospital after two weeks and had fully recovered six weeks after the infection.

E. Bundibugyo Ebolavirus (BDBV)

On November 24, 2007, the Uganda Ministry of Health confirmed an outbreak of Ebola in the Bundibugyo District. After confirmation of samples tested by the United States National Reference Laboratories and the CDC, the World Health Organization confirmed the presence of the new species. On 20 February 2008, the Uganda Ministry officially announced the epidemic in Bundibugyo, ending with the last infected person discharged on 8 January 2008. An epidemiological study conducted by WHO and scientists from the Uganda Ministry of Health, determined that there were 116confirmed and probable cases of the new

Ebola species, and that the outbreak had a mortality rate of 34%.

As already indicated before, the genera Ebola virus and Marburgvirus were originally classified as the species of the now-obsolete genus Filo virus. But In March 1998, the Vertebrate Virus Subcommittee suggested. In the International Committee on Taxonomy of Viruses (ICTV) to change the genus Filovirus to the family Filoviridae with two specific genera: Ebola- like viruses and Marburg-like viruses. This proposal was implemented in Washington, D.C., as of April 2001 and in Paris as of July 2002. In 2000, another proposal was made in Washington, D.C., and that was to change the suffix “like viruses” to “-virus”, resulting in today’s “Ebolavirus” and “Marburgvirus.”

The Marburg virus causes hemorrhagic fever in humans and non-human.

Chapter 4B/1

The Marburg viruses

The Marburg virus causes hemorrhagic fever in humans and non-human.

Scientists identified Marburg virus in 1967, when small outbreaks occurred among lab workers in Marburg, which is a town and a tourist attraction situated in the central part of west central Germany. The lab workers were exposed to infected monkeys imported from Uganda. Marburg virus is like Ebola in that both can cause hemorrhagic fever, meaning that infected people develop high fevers and bleeding throughout the body that can lead to shock, organ failure and death.

Chapter 5/1

The life cycle of the Dengue virus

Dengue viruses are transmitted to humans by the bite of an infected mosquito. The Dengue fever virus first appeared in the 1950s in the Philippines and Thailand and has since spread throughout the tropical and subtropical regions of the globe. Up to 40% of the world's population now lives in areas where the dengue virus is endemic, and the disease — with the mosquitoes that carry it — is likely to spread farther as the world warms.

According to WHO, Dengue virus infects 50 to 100 million people per year. The virus has a mortality rate of 2.5 percent which is lower than some other viruses, virus can cause an Ebola-like disease that is called "dengue hemorrhagic fever" and this condition has a mortality rate of 20%, if left untreated.

A vaccine for Dengue was approved in 2019 by the U.S. Food and Drug Administration for children of 9-16 years old living in an area where dengue is common and has a confirmed history of virus infection. In some countries, an approved vaccine is available for those 9-45 years old, but again, recipients must have contracted a confirmed case of dengue in the past. Those who have not caught the virus before, could be put at risk of developing severe dengue if given the vaccine.

As already indicated, Dengue is a mosquito-borne viral infection causing a severe flu-like illness. Sometimes the virus causes causing a potentially lethal complication called "severe dengue." Half of the world's population is at risk, and it affects infants, young children, and adults. The incidence dengue has increased as 30-fold over the last 50 years. Upto50-100 million infections are now estimated to occur annually in over one hundred endemic countries, putting almost half of the world's population at risk. Bangladesh is one of the countries that are affected by virus.

The Aedes aegypti mosquito is the main vector that transmits the virus. The virus is passed to humans through the bites of an infective female Aedes mosquito, which acquired the virus while feeding on the blood fan infected person.

As already indicated, once humans are infected, they become the main carriers and multipliers of the virus and serve as a source of the virus for uninfected mosquitoes. The virus circulates in the blood of an infected person for 2 to 7 days. At this period, the person develops a fever. Patients who are already infected with the dengue virus can transmit the infection via Aedes mosquitoes after the first symptoms appear (normally within 4 to 5 days to a maximum of 12 days).

The clinical features of dengue fever vary according to the age of the patient. Dengue fever normally causes high fever (40°C/ 104°F) and at least two of these following symptoms:

Severe headaches, pain behind the eyes, nausea, vomiting, swollen glands, muscle and joint pains and rash.

In humans, recovery from infection by one dengue viruses provides lifelong immunity against that virus' serotype. However, this immunity confers only partial and transient protection against subsequent infection by the other three serotypes of the viruses.

In the meantime, here are some practical tips to minimize the breeding of Aedes aegypti mosquitoes within our community.

Environmental management: Changing the environment by destroying, altering, removing, or recycling non-essential containers to minimize and/ or prevent mosquito from breeding. This can help to minimize the vector propagation and human contact with vector-pathogens.

Mosquito-proofing of water-storage containers: Water tank storage can serve as larval habitats. Yet, it can be designed to prevent mosquitoes from laying its egg on the surface of water by having fitted tight lids. If rain-filled, tightly fitted mesh screens allow the rainwater to be harvested while keeping mosquitoes out. Moreover, removable cover should be replaced regularly and well-maintained to prevent damage which then allows mosquitoes to have access to the water tank.

Solid waste management: In the context of dengue vector control, 'solid-waste' refers to non-biodegradable items of household or community. A proper storage, collection and disposal of waste are especially important. Therefore, "reduce, reuse and recycle" principle must be universally applicable to reduce larval habitats.

Street cleansing: A regular street cleaning, including removing discarded water-bearing containers and cleaning drainage water is incredibly significant act to prevent mosquitoes from breeding.

Personal's prevention: (1) wearing light-colored clothes; (2) installing mosquito net on doors and windows; (3) hanging the mosquito net over the sleeping area. It is be noted that Aedes mosquitoes tend to bite during the day. Keep patients under a bed net to prevent Aedes mosquitoes spreading the viruses to healthy people.

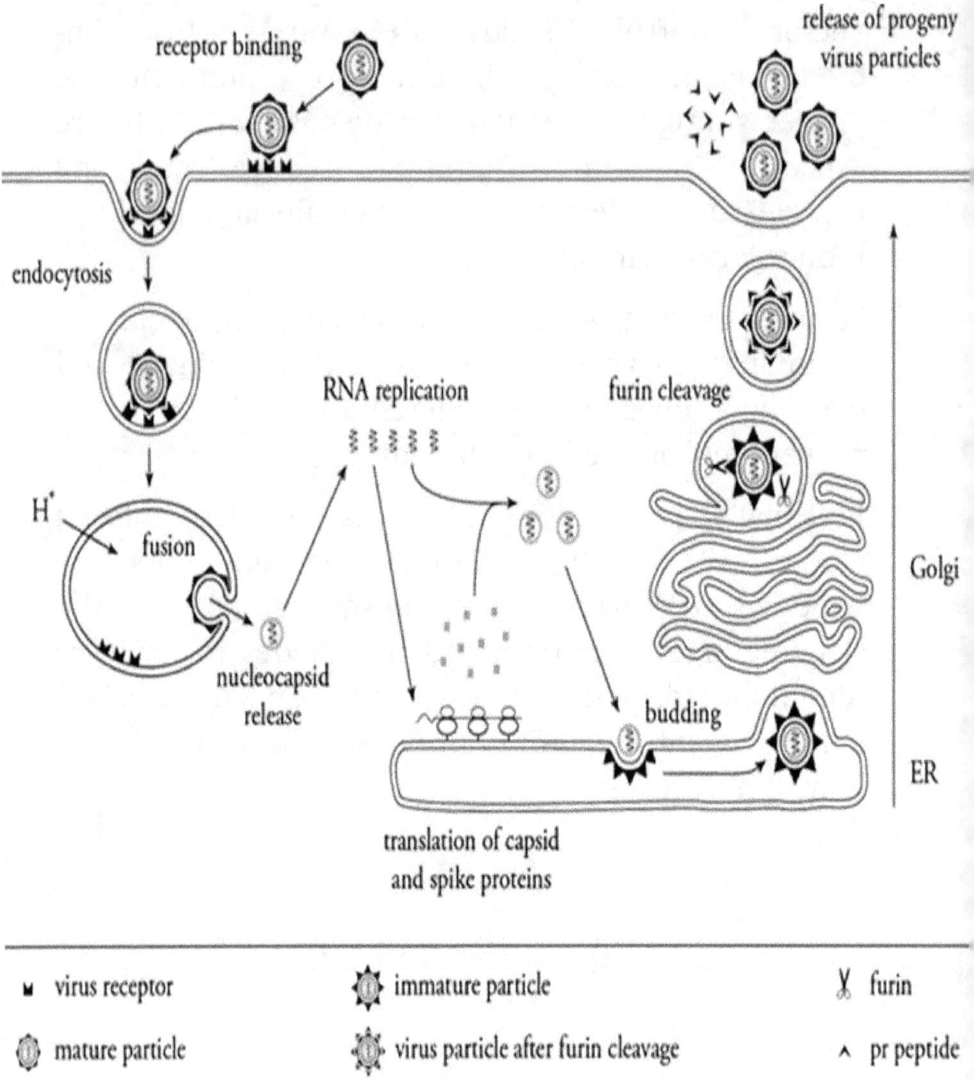

Dengue virus is an RNA virus. Its outer surface is covered with envelope proteins surrounding a lipid bilayer envelope. Inside the envelope is a capsid shell that contains the virus's RNA genome. The Dengue virus infects immune cells.

There are two cell surface receptor molecules important in dengue infection. The cognate receptor[36]) is involved in normal infections and the CF receptor is involved in the phenomenon called "antibody dependent enhancement."

The virus' envelope protein binds to the cognate receptor and triggers a cellular process called "receptor-mediated endometriosis[37]). The virus is internalized in a bubble-like structure called the endoscope.

When endoscopes form, proton pumps[38]) lower the pH of the interior. The virus responds to the lowered pH by changing the conformation of the envelope proteins to form spike-like structures.

The tips of the spikes are hydrophobic, which allows them to penetrate someone's membrane. (a uterine membrane). They bend until someone's membrane and the virus's membrane fuse together and release the

---

[36] *Cognate - related; connected; associated; · allied; · interconnected; · linked; · coupled.*

[37] *Receptor mediated endometriosis – in the uterus, estrogen receptor beta plays a critical role in endometriosis (an inflammation of the uterus' lining).*

[38] *Proton pump - H+ pumps are located primarily in the luminal membranes of the mitochondria-rich α-intercalated cells. There are two major H+ pumps in this segment, an H+-ATPase and an H+/K+-ATPase, the former is particularly important for an acid–base condition*

capsid into the cytoplasm. The capsid breaks apart and releases the viral RNA.

The viral RNA travels to the rough endoplasmic reticulum. It is a positive-sense strand and can be directly translated into proteins. The ends of the RNA form structure that binds to translation initiation proteins. The complex attaches to the ribosomes to initiate translation. The whole viral genome is translated as a single, long, polyprotein chain. The capsid protein is on the cytoplasm side of the endoplasmic reticulum. The envelope protein and the membrane protein are in the lumen side and are activated by the host's peptidase enzyme.

In the cytoplasm, one of the viral proteins, a protease enzyme, activates all the other proteins in the poly protein chain. These proteins aggregate to form the RNA replication complex.

Viral RNA is synthesized in multiple steps. First, the ends of the viral RNA fold up, and the RNA forms a circle. The RNA then attaches to the replication complex to start the first round of synthesis. Using the RNA's positive-sense RNA as a template a negative- sense copy is made. The pair of RNA strands forms a double helix.

The RNA then becomes a circle again. This time the negative-sense strand acts as a template to make a positive-sense strand. Many copies of the positive- sense RNA strand is made by repeated cycles of RNA synthesis. Some of these strands are translated to make more viral proteins. Eventually enough proteins are made to assemble new viruses.

The envelope proteins aggregate in the lumen of the endoplasmic reticulum and the capsid protein segregate on the cytoplasmic side. A viral RNA binds to the capsid protein and is packaged into a new virus particle as it buds off into the endoplasmic reticulum. The virus is still immature. Its pre-membrane proteins cover the tips of the envelope proteins to prevent premature fusion back into the cell. The virus buds off and travels through the Golgi apparatus and continues toward the cell surface. Before reaching the surface, the pre-membrane protein is processed, and a virus becomes mature. New dengue viruses are released from the cell ready to infect other cells.

Note that the scheme containing the life cycle of the Dengue virus describe all the steps up until the virus' maturation.

Chapter 6/1

Protection of babies by vaccines.

Two vaccines are now available to protect children from rotavirus, the leading cause of severe diarrheal illness among babies and young children. The virus can spread rapidly, through what researchers call the fecal-oral route (meaning that small particles of feces end up being consumed).

An oral vaccine against rotavirus infection is given to babies as part of their routine childhood vaccinations.

The vaccine is given as two doses, 4 weeks apart. Usually, the first dose is given at 8 weeks, and the second dose at 12 weeks. The vaccine is given as a liquid straight into the baby's mouth for them to swallow. The vaccine is a weakened virus.

Although children in the developed world rarely die from rotavirus infection, the disease is a killer in the developing world, where rehydration treatments are not widely available.

The WHO estimates that worldwide, 453,000 children younger than age 5 died from rotavirus infection in 2008. But countries that have introduced the vaccine have reported sharp declines in rotavirus hospitalizations and deaths.

Chapter 7/1

Epidemiology of the measles virus and its vaccines

Measles (also called Rubeola) is a highly contagious, serious disease. Before the introduction of measles vaccine in 1963 and widespread vaccination, major epidemics occurred approximately every 2–3 years and measles caused an estimated 2.6 million deaths each year. Even though a safe and cost-effective vaccine is now available, in 2018, there were more than 140 000 measles deaths globally, mostly among children under the age of five. However, measles vaccination resulted in a 73% drop in measles deaths between 2000 and 2018 worldwide!!

In 2018, about 86% of the world's children received one dose of measles vaccine by their first birthday through routine health services – up from 72% in 2000.

During 2000- 2018, measles vaccination prevented an estimated 23.2 million deaths making measles one of the best vaccines in public health!

Still, more than 140 000 people died from measles in 2018 – mostly children under the age of 5years, despite the availability of a safe and defective vaccine.

Chapter 7/2

Structure of the measles virus

Measles virus called also Morbilli0 is the prototypic) member of the Morbillivirus genus of the family Paramyxoviridae.

The virus is spherical with a diameter, ranging from 100 to 300 nm and has two major structural components: one is the helical ribonucleoprotein (RNP) core formed by the association of the nucleoprotein (N), the phosphoprotein (P) and the large protein (L) with the viral genome. The other major component is the cellular membrane-derived lipid envelope surrounding the RNP core.

The measles virus has two glycoproteins spikes that play a significant role in pathogenesis: F (fusion) protein spikes and the H (haemagglutinin) protein spikes.

Fusion proteins are responsible for the fusion of the virus with host cell membranes and viral penetration.

Haemagglutinin proteins are responsible for the binding of the virus to cells, and they are the antigens against which neutralizing antibodies are formed.

Following is a scheme of the measles virus:

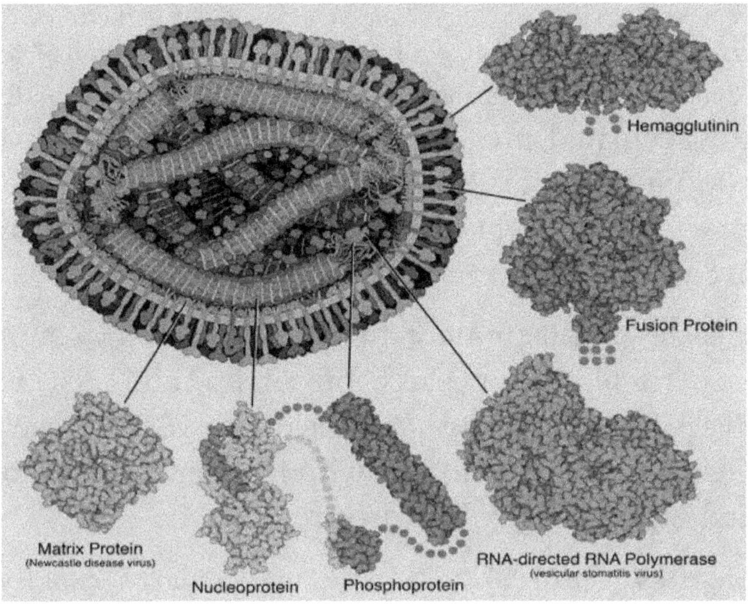

Signs and symptoms

The first sign of measles is usually a high fever, which begins about 10 to 12 days after exposure to the virus and lasts 4 to 7 days. A runny nose, a cough, red and watery eyes, and small white spots inside the cheeks can develop in the initial stage. After several days, a rash erupts, usually on the face and upper neck. Over about 3 days, the rash spreads, eventually reaching the hands and feet. The rash lasts for 5 to 6 days, and then fades. On average, the rash occurs 14 days after exposure to the virus (within a range of 7 to 18 days).

Who is at risk?

Unvaccinated young children are at highest risk of measles and its complications, including death. Unvaccinated pregnant women are also at risk. Any non-immune person (who has not been vaccinated or was vaccinated but did not develop immunity) can become infected.

Measles is still common in many developing countries – particularly in parts of Africa and Asia. The overwhelming majority (more than 95%) of measles deaths occur in countries with low per capita incomes and weak health infrastructures.

Measles outbreaks can be particularly deadly in countries experiencing or recovering from a natural disaster or conflict. Damage to health infrastructure and health services interrupts routine immunization and overcrowding in residential camps increases the risk of infection.

Transmission

Measles is one of the world's most contagious diseases. It is spread by coughing and sneezing, close personal contact, or direct contact with infected nasal or throat secretions.

The virus remains active and contagious in the air or on infected surfaces for up to 2 hours. It can be transmitted by an infected person from 4 days prior to the onset of the rash to 4 days after the rash erupts.

Measles outbreak scan result in epidemics that cause many deaths, especially among young, malnourished children. In countries where measles has been eliminated, cases imported from other countries remain an important source of infection.

Chapter 7/3

The replication cycle of the measles Virus

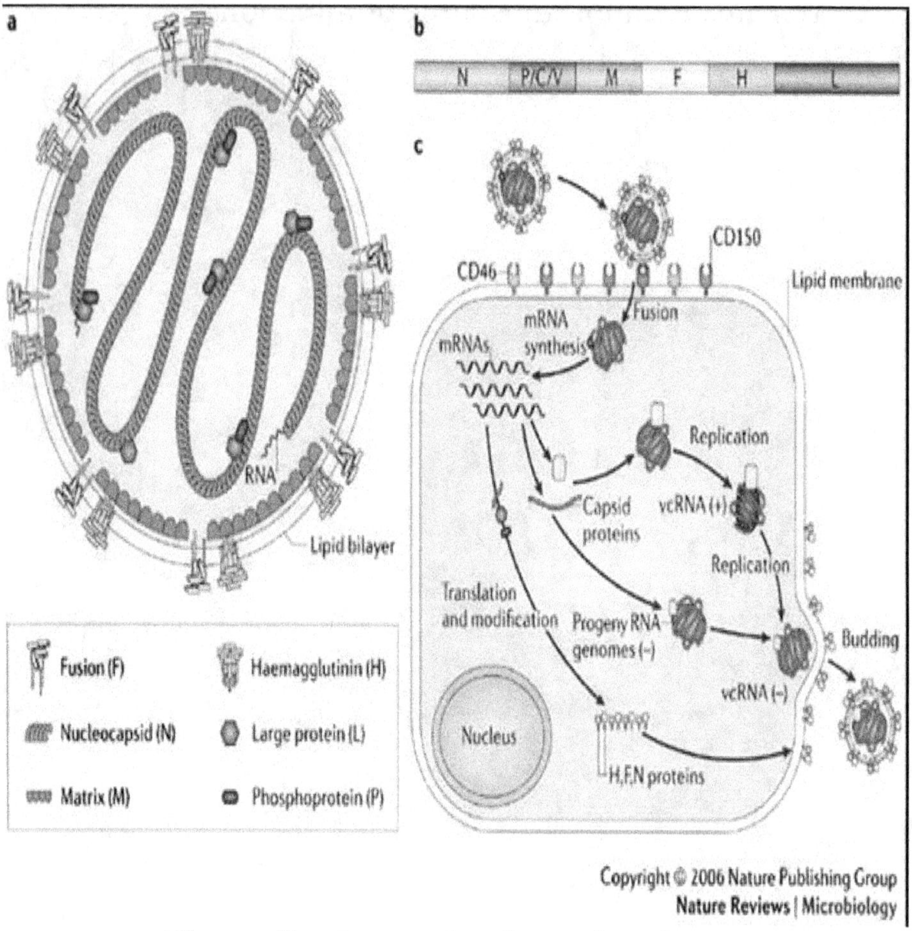

The replication cycle of measles virus

The Hemagglutinin (H) protein spikes and the Fusion (F) protein spikes mediate transmission of the measles virus into host cells in the human respiratory tract. The virus is absorbed into the host cells when the Hemagglutinin protein spikes bind to the CD46 and CD150 host cellular receptors. Once uncoated in the host cell, RNA polymerase transcribes the viral RNA genome into mRNA, which then undergoes translation to manufacture viral proteins. These viral proteins function to formulate new helical capsids for the replication of the virus, which eventually leaves the host cell through the process of budding. Although the transmission of the virus initially infects the upper respiratory tract, replication of the virus in Epithelial cells can spread the virus to the lymph nodes and further replication in the lymphatic system can spread the virus to other organs including the liver, skin, kidneys, and gastrointestinal tract, virus-infects human epithelial cells, endothelial cells, and macrophages.

The virus' mode of infection is airborne droplets and can be transmitted by exposure to someone infected with this pathogen. The measles is exceedingly infectious and transmitted by respiratory fluid secretions most commonly from sneezing or coughing.

The end

www.ingramcontent.com/pod-product-compliance
Lightning Source LLC
LaVergne TN
LVHW011936070526
838202LV00054B/4682